OXFORD MEDICAL PUBLICATIONS

Multiple Sclerosis Care

Published and forthcoming Oxford Care Manuals

Stroke Care: A Practical Manual
Rowan Harwood, Farhad Huwez, and Dawn Good

Multiple Sclerosis Care: A Practical Manual
John Zajicek, Jennifer Freeman, and Bernadette Porter

Dementia Care: A Practical Manual
Jonathan Waite, Rowan Harwood, Ian Morton, and David Connelly

Headache: A Practical Manual
David Kernick and Peter Goadsby (eds)

Diabetes Care: A Practical Manual
Rowan Hillson

Oxford Care Manuals
Multiple Sclerosis Care: A Practical Manual

John Zajicek
Consultant Neurologist,
Derriford Hospital Plymouth;
Chair, Clinical Neuroscience,
Peninsula Medical School, Plymouth, UK

Jennifer Freeman
Reader in Physiotherapy and Rehabilitation,
School of Allied Health,
Faculty of Health and Social Work,
Plymouth University;
Honorary Lecturer, Institute of Neurology,
London, UK

and

Bernadette Porter
Nurse Consultant—Multiple Sclerosis,
National Hospital for Neurology and Neurosurgery,
UCLH Trust, London, UK

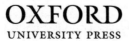

OXFORD
UNIVERSITY PRESS

OXFORD
UNIVERSITY PRESS

Great Clarendon Street, Oxford OX2 6DP

Oxford University Press is a department of the University of Oxford.
It furthers the University's objective of excellence in research, scholarship,
and education by publishing worldwide in

Oxford New York

Auckland Cape Town Dar es Salaam Hong Kong Karachi
Kuala Lumpur Madrid Melbourne Mexico City Nairobi
New Delhi Shanghai Taipei Toronto

With offices in

Argentina Austria Brazil Chile Czech Republic France Greece
Guatemala Hungary Italy Japan Poland Portugal Singapore
South Korea Switzerland Thailand Turkey Ukraine Vietnam

Oxford is a registered trade mark of Oxford University Press
in the UK and in certain other countries

Published in the United States
by Oxford University Press Inc., New York

© Oxford University Press, 2007

The moral rights of the authors have been asserted
Database right Oxford University Press (maker)

First published 2007

British Library Cataloguing in Publication Data
Data available

Library of Congress Cataloging in Publication Data
Data available

Typeset by Newgen Imaging Systems (P) Ltd., Chennai, India
Printed in Great Britain
on acid-free paper by
Clays Ltd., Bungay, Suffolk

ISBN 978–0–19–856983–1 (Pbk: alk. paper)

1

Preface

Multiple sclerosis (MS) is a complex chronic neurological condition that not only affects directly the lives of those with it, but can also impact on family members, friends, and work colleagues. The potential psychosocial impact of the disease can be more burdensome than its physical consequences. Help to deal with these problems is best provided in the context of an experienced multidisciplinary team, and an understanding of the diagnosis and its implications by health and social service professionals can greatly assist people to cope with the wider impacts of MS.

We have written this handbook with the specific intention of making it accessible to everyone involved in providing care for people with MS, and also hope that people with MS themselves may find some relevance in some sections. As doctor, physiotherapist, and nurse, we hope that we have provided different perspectives on the management of MS, so that information can be accessed quickly and efficiently. We hope that the book will be helpful for general practitioners, nurses, junior doctors, consultants, therapists of all description, social workers, carers, and other interested professionals.

We make no apology for concentrating on some aspects not normally covered in conventional texts, including details on measurement instruments, clinical trials, and other research-related issues. It is only by measurement that we will know whether what we do as health and social care professionals really has an impact in helping people with MS, and the measurement message is becoming increasingly adopted as we seek to improve lives.

The message from people with MS has been very strong—a cure is wanted, but people also want ways of improving day-to-day living in order to minimize the impact of MS. A cure will only come with everyone working in partnership—health and social staff, charities, carers, and people with MS—as well as everyone having the chance to participate in research if they wish. We hope this book will provide information about how to improve people's lives with practical suggestions in the short-term, but also encourage people to understand and take part in research, which we all hope will find a cure in the not too distant future.

JZ, JF, BP
January 2007

Contents

Part 4 Ongoing management

Part 5 Evaluation of services

Part 6 Useful resources

Detailed contents

Abbreviations

2-AG	2-arachidonoylglycerol
ADEM	acute disseminated encephalomyelitis
AFO	ankle foot orthoses
ASA	aryl-sulphatase A
BBB	blood–brain–barrier
BI	Barthel Index
CAMS	cannabinoids in MS
CDMS	clinically definite MS
CHI	Commission for Health Improvement
CIS	clinically isolated syndromes
CISC	clean, intermittent self-catheterization
CNS	central nervous system
CSF	cerebrospinal fluid
CUPID	cannabinoid use in progressive inflammatory brain disease
DDC	demyelinating disease diagnostic clinic
DDAVP	desmopressin
DWI	diffusion weighted imaging
EAE	experimental allergic encephalomyelitis
EDSS	expanded disability status scale
ESIMS	European Study on Immunoglobulin in MS
ETOMS	early treatment of multiple sclerosis with Rebif®
FES	functional electrical simulation
FIM	functional independence measure
FSS	fatigue severity scale
FSS	functional systems scales
GalC	galactocerebroside beta galactosidase gene
gd-DTPA	gadolinium DTPA
GNDS	Guy's Neurological Disability Scale (renamed the UK Neurological Disability Scale)
ICF	World Health Organization's International Classification of Functioning, Disability and Health
ICP	integrated care pathway
IFN	interferon
IFN-β	interferon-beta
IFN-γ	interferon-gamma
IgG	immunoglobulin
INO	internuclear ophthalmoplegia

IVIg	intravenous immunoglobulins
LHON	Leber's Hereditary Optic Neuropathy
LMN	lower motor neuron
LOD	logarithm of the odds
LR	lateral rectus
MDEM	multiphasic disseminated encephalomyelitis
MFIS	modified fatigue impact scale
MHC	major histocompatibility complex
MIU	million international units
MLF	medial longitudinal fasiculus
MR	medial rectus
MRI	magnetic resonance imaging
MRS	magnetic resonance spectroscopy
MS	multiple sclerosis
MSCRG	MS Collaborative Research Group
MSFC	multiple sclerosis functional composite
MSIS-29	multiple sclerosis impact scale
MSQOL-54	multiple sclerosis quality of life-54 instrument
MSSS-88	Multiple Sclerosis Spasticity Scale
MSWS-12	12-item multiple sclerosis walking scale
MTR	magnetization transfer ratio
NHS	UK National Health Service
NICE	National Institute of Clinical Excellence
NMO	neuromyelitis optica
NSF	National Service Framework
NZB	natalizumab
OWIMS	once weekly interferon for MS study group
PASAT	paced auditory serial addition test
PEG	percutaneous gastronomy
PLP	proteolipid protein
PML	progressive multifocal leucoencephalopathy
PPMS	primary progressive MS
PRISMS	Preventions of Relapses and Disability by IFNβ -1a in MS Study Group
PWMS	people with multiple sclerosis
RIMS	rehabilitation in multiple sclerosis
RRMS	relapsing-remitting phase of MS
SCA	spino-cerebellar ataxias
SF-36	the Medical Outcome Study Short Form-36
SLE	systematic lupus erythematosus
SPECTRIMS	Secondary Progressive Efficacy Clinical Trial of Rebif® (IFN-β 1a) in MS
SPMS	secondary progressive MS

SWIMS	South West Impact of MS study
TENS	transcutaneous electrical nerve simulation
TPMT	thiopurine methyl transferase
UKNDS	UK Neurological Disabilty Scale
UMN	upper motor neuron
VCAM-1	vascular cell adhesion molecule-1
VEP	visual evoked potential
VER	visual evoked response
X-ALD	X-linked adrenoleukodystrophy

Part 1

Background

The history of multiple sclerosis (MS)

Earliest history of MS

The earliest recorded historical descriptions of diseases can help in providing clues about causes of those diseases. Good evidence for the recorded presence of MS is lacking prior to the mid nineteenth century. The first clinical evidence probably occurs in the grandson of King George III in 1822. Pathological descriptions then appeared in the 1830s, from Cruveilhier in France, and Carswell in England. However, most credit for the detailed descriptions of both clinical and pathological aspects of MS goes to Jean Martin Charcot, from the Salpetriere in Paris towards the end of that century. Charcot's descriptions of *sclerose en plaques* remain seminal to this day, and indeed some of his writings, particularly around the involvement of loss of nerve cell processes (axons) in the pathology of the condition, have been neglected until relatively recently.

Structure of the nervous system

At the same time as the pathology of MS was being described, advances were being made in our understanding of how the nervous system is constituted. Virchow (1858) believed that the nervous system was composed of neurons and neuroglia—or nerve glue. It was not until Cajal (1913) and Hortega (1921) that specific components of the supporting cell structure were identified. The major types of glial cells are the **astrocytes** (which have various functions including maintenance of the barrier between blood and brain, keeping the ionic environment stable, and scar formation), and **oligodendrocytes** (which produce and maintain the myelin sheaths surrounding nerves in the central nervous system, allowing fast nerve conduction to occur). Loss of myelin (**demyelination**) and oligodendrocytes, with inflammation and astrocyte overgrowth are features of MS.

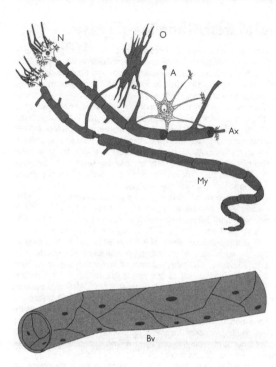

Fig. 1.1 The normal central nervous system is largely composed of neurons (N), extending axonal processes (Ax), which are insulated by processes from oligo-dendrocytes (O). Each oligodendrocyte may extend between 30–50 individual processes, each in turn supporting a segment of compact myelin, which facilitates fast electrical conduction. In normal tissue, astrocytes (A) have many functions, including extending processes to natural gaps between the myelin segments, known as nodes of Ranvier. They also help to maintain the balance of sodium and potassium and contribute to maintaining the normally tight barrier between blood and brain in blood vessels (Bv).

Phases of describing the disease

Different pathological variants of what appears to be the same underlying demyelinating inflammatory disease were described around the turn of the twentieth century. These included Devic's neuromyelitis optica (1894), Marburg's hyperacute disease (1906), Schilder's variant (1912), and Balo's concentric sclerosis (1928).

It was Charcot's view that overgrowth of the supporting glial cells strangled the insulating myelin sheath, sometimes leading to death of axons, with secondary blood vessel changes. James Dawson (1916) placed greater emphasis on the role of inflammation centred around blood vessels, the so-called 'Dawson's fingers' of inflammatory cells around venules in the brain. He clearly described inflammation, demyelination, and various stages of development of the plaque. Over the years, theories were produced associating MS with toxins or infections, and such theories continue to circulate today. However, as new technologies and new areas of science have emerged, theories about the cause of MS have altered. Although Charcot described the occurrence of MS in families, it was not really until after the Second World War that epidemiological studies of MS really gathered speed. These suggested that environmental exposure at an early age in genetically predisposed individuals may precipitate MS. Similarly, the development of immunology in the 1960s and 1970s, together with advances in genetics, led to increased evidence for development of the autoimmune hypothesis of MS. Although the first animal models of demyelination were described in the 1930s following rabies vaccination, the development of these models in the 1970s, heavily influenced the debate regarding pathogenesis and treatment. The 1980s brought the development of magnetic resonance scanning, which has revolutionized our understanding of diagnosis, and has coincided with the emergence of large randomized controlled trials of treatments.

Inflammation and demyelination in the central nervous system, described by many of the authors above, are undoubtedly hallmarks of MS. However, these findings do not provide clear clues about the cause of MS, as most tissue obtained for pathological evaluation over the years has been obtained from chronic MS cases. These cases may not reflect initial pathological processes, indeed recent pathological studies have suggested possible alternative explanations in a search for the cause of MS.

In discussing these issues with people affected by MS, we do well to maintain an open mind. Historians study history as it can teach us a lot that may be of relevance to living in the twenty-first century. In science, old ideas are often recirculated as new technologies emerge, and although there is a great tendency to pin hopes on the latest theory or treatment option, we still do not know the cause of MS and are even further from a cure.

Chapter 2

MS pathology

Plaques and relapsing-remitting MS

The hallmark of MS pathology is the plaque, as originally described by Charcot. People often refer to such affected areas within the central nervous system (CNS) as **lesions**, which is a more generic term for any area of abnormality. The term **sclerosis** means hardening, derived from early studies where brains from people with MS were found to contain areas of hardened, scarred tissue.

Early plaque development appears to be focused around small blood vessels, often around the ventricles within the brain (peri-ventricular), and is composed of cellular infiltration and breakdown of the normally tight blood–brain barrier (BBB). The cell infiltrate is mostly T-lymphocyte, with B-lymphocyte and macrophage involvement as well. There is some controversy about the relationship between BBB breakdown and demyelination, but the two events do appear to be associated. Most of the myelin breakdown seems to be conducted by macrophages, which are the only cell type consistently seen in association with myelin. Studies using MRI have demonstrated lesions occurring much more frequently than clinical episodes (or relapses), and the likelihood of any episode becoming clinically obvious is related to the site and size of the lesions.

Recovery from any episode seems to be associated with a reduction in the cellular infiltrate, a restoration of the integrity of the BBB, and a degree of myelin repair. Such repair can be seen pathologically as a 'shadow plaque', where the myelin is thinner than usual, as new myelin is laid down. Research into what factors control myelin repair is very active and we would dearly like to know why some people seem able to sustain multiple episodes of inflammatory attack with little apparent disability, whereas others fail to mount a repair response. Some of this explanation may lie in the quantity of nerve cell damage (both to axons and nerve cell bodies), and astrocytic scarring which follows any single episode of damage. Recent studies have re-emphasised Charcot's observations concerning the importance of early axonal transection in acute plaques, and many people have used this as a rationale for early introduction of immuno-modulatory drugs to reduce the risk of subsequent nerve damage. As far as we are aware, any loss of nerves within the central nervous system is likely to be permanent, as mammalian nervous systems have lost the ability to regenerate, unlike some other cell systems such as skin or bone. Again, this is an area of active research, particularly as precursor cells seemingly able to differentiate into nerve and glial cells have not only been identified in mammalian nervous systems, but also in bone marrow.

Progressive MS

Unfortunately, a large proportion of people with MS will go on to develop significant disability. This is due to damage accumulation during acute relapses (from nerve cell damage and scar tissue formation), but also due to transition from the relapsing-remitting phase of MS (RRMS), into a more progressive phase (so-called secondary progressive). Most people's MS will start with episodes, in the form of RRMS, but the majority will probably go on to develop secondary progressive disease. About 15% of people will start their disease with a primary progressive course. There are some differences in the pathologies of these different phases of the condition. Primary progressive disease tends to involve the spinal cord more severely, with relative sparing of the brain. The pathology of secondary progressive MS reflects the chronicity of the inflammatory process, and most of the classical descriptions have been derived from such patients. Plaques can be of varying age, with evidence of new inflammation often mixed with scarring and areas of complete demyelination.

New studies of MS pathology

In an attempt to investigate the earliest possible events in the MS inflammatory cascade of damage and repair, researchers have tried to look more closely at tissue obtained from people in the earliest stages of MS, often because they died unexpectedly or had biopsies where there has been clinical doubt about the diagnosis. Critics may say that these cases may not represent typical cases of MS, but the results have yielded some very interesting findings. There appears to be much more of a role for programmed cell death (apoptosis) in at least some of these cases. Some investigators maintain that these processes in oligodendrocytes may be the primary phenomenon in the majority of cases, so that inflammation may be secondary to cell death (for whatever reason). Others have identified four different pathological types, with all lesions in any one individual being of the same type. The first two types are predominantly inflammatory, and the latter two types mainly associated with cell death. These studies may have profound implications for our understanding of the disease; if inflammation may be a secondary phenomenon in at least some cases, possibly with more progressive clinical courses, then this would influence treatment regimens.

Another view starting to emerge from a variety of sources is that not all inflammation may be bad. Most inflammation that occurs in our bodies aims to assist in repair processes, and although we currently believe that MS is predominantly an autoimmune disease with overactive inflammation, there is evidence emerging to suggest that inflammation can sometimes be useful in repairing the nervous system. Treatments targeted at blocking factors that experimental evidence would suggest should be bad for CNS damage can sometimes make things worse, and conversely, introducing some types of inflammation can assist in repair. We await further research in these areas with great interest.

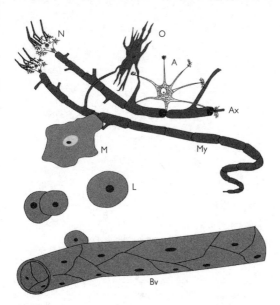

Fig. 2.1 In MS, the normally tight blood–brain barrier becomes more permeable, with passage of inflammatory cells, particularly lymphocytes (L) into the brain substance. This stimulates the immune system to initiate inflammatory attack on myelin (My), mostly through macrophages and microglia (M), leading to loss of myelin, reduced nerve conduction and loss of the myelin-forming oligodendrocytes (O). With repeated episodes of inflammation, there is progressive loss of nerve cells (N), and overgrowth of astrocytes (A), causing scar tissue to form.

Immunology of MS

Basic immunology

The immune system is broadly divided into two main arms: cellular immunity—where specific cells (mostly T-lymphocytes or T-cells) implement the immune response, and humoral immunity—where antibodies produced by B-lymphocytes (or B-cells) are the major effector mechanism. The immune response is directed against antigens on the surface of foreign cells, or components of foreign cells that are broken down and presented to T-cells at the T-cell receptor. Most cells in our bodies contain surface markers or antigens that enable cells and antibodies of our own immune system to recognize our own cells as 'self', thereby avoiding attack from our own immune system. These cell surface markers are divided into class I and class II molecules, whose expression is determined by genes in the major histocompatibility complex (MHC) on chromosome 6. This lack of response to self-antigens is known as self-tolerance, and autoimmune diseases may occur when tolerance to self-antigens fails. The immune system is extremely complex, with multiple signalling processes occurring all the time. These signals may be mediated both by direct contact between cells (by cell surface molecules including adhesion molecules and T-cell receptors), and also by molecules secreted by neighbouring cells (including compounds such as cytokines and lymphokines). T-cells are at the centre of the immune response, and the interaction between T-cells and cells that present antigen at the T-cell receptor is sometimes referred to as the immunological synapse (see Fig. 3.1). Most components of this interaction are being tested as potential treatments in MS.

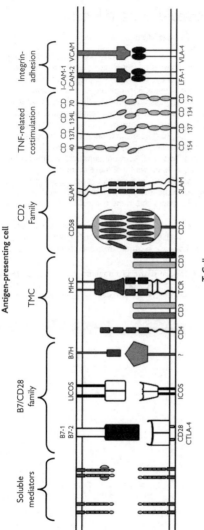

Fig. 3.1 The immunological synapse in more detail.

Reasons for considering MS as an autoimmune disease

Most people believe that MS is an autoimmune disease, with the body's own defences targeted against myelin. There are several lines of evidence implicating an overactive immune system in the pathogenesis of MS:

- Pathological studies showing influx of lymphocytes around blood vessels, associated with demyelination, compatible with autoimmunity.
- Experimental animal models can be produced (experimental allergic encephalomyelitis (EAE) whereby it is possible to immunize animals with components of myelin, so that an autoimmune inflammatory response can be induced, with pathology similar to human MS. Some models are better than others, and there are considerable limitations to the conclusions that can be drawn from these models.
- Genetic studies show associations with certain genetic types (so-called polymorphisms) involved in the immune response, most notably certain genes in the MHC, important in the control of the immune response.
- Family studies have shown increased incidence of other autoimmune diseases such as diabetes mellitus, pernicious anaemia, thyroid disease and inflammatory bowel disease in other family members as well as in people affected by MS.

Against the autoimmune theory is the fact that no one has ever been able to transfer any factor from people with MS into animals to cause a similar condition, and no specific target antigen has ever been identified on myelin.

MS definitions and disease classification

Clinical terms

Although the precise criteria by which a diagnosis of MS can be made have changed over the years, the essential clinical criteria remain: evidence for episodes of inflammation in different parts of the nervous system at different times. In other words, there should be evidence for dissemination of lesions in both time and place within the central nervous system, with exclusion of any alternative explanations.

Most people will start their MS with episodes of neurological dysfunction attributable to a problem in the central nervous system. At first presentation these are known as **clinically isolated syndromes** (CIS), as one cannot be certain whether any individual person will go on to develop further episodes, and hence have a confirmed clinical diagnosis of MS. Once further episodes have occurred, a person will be labelled as having **RRMS**, which is the commonest presenting form of the condition in around 85% of cases.

The definition of a **relapse** is conventionally an episode of neurological dysfunction attributable to a lesion within the central nervous system (either when new symptoms develop or existing ones deteriorate), lasting for at least 24 hours, not attributable to fever and with objective evidence from examination for a change, against a stable clinical background of at least a month. In reality these definitions are rather arbitrary, and evidence from studies using MRI have demonstrated ongoing inflammatory brain activity often in the absence of any clinical change. Such definitions are usually created to satisfy criteria in clinical trials, whereas clinical experience tells us that people with MS often experience episodes of temporary deterioration, perhaps with an increase in fatigue, but with little to find on neurological examination. This reflects more on our inability to detect change using conventional clinical examination techniques, and much more work is needed on the definition of a relapse from the perspective of the person affected by the condition.

The rate of relapse in MS varies according to age and population studied, but approximate rate is around one relapse every 1–2 years (using the definition outlined above). There is some debate over how long a relapse can persist before established disability is permanent, but there is evidence for recovery from relapses up to at least 6 months after acute deterioration, and sometimes much longer. This fact can offer hope to patients, but can interfere with the interpretation of clinical trials when permanent disability (often called progression) has sometimes been defined as deterioration on two consecutive clinic visits only 3 months apart.

Unfortunately, with time, the majority of people who start with RRMS will change into a more insidious progressive course—**secondary progressive MS** (SPMS). This would be unusual until at least three years after diagnosis, and about 50% of people may be in this phase after 10 years (see Chapter 9, Natural history studies). In practical terms it is very difficult to say prospectively whether someone is going be in this phase of the condition, and it is really only possible to use this label after someone has gone through at least 12 months of progressive deterioration.

About 10–15% of people may present with a progressive clinical deterioration from the start of their problems—**primary progressive MS** (PPMS). Such individuals tend to be a little older on presentation and have a more equal sex incidence, whereas RRMS and SPMS are commoner in women by about 2:1. Presenting with PPMS can make diagnosis more difficult as other conditions need to be considered (see Chapter 11, Diagnosis).

Different sets of **diagnostic criteria** have been produced over the years. The Schumacher criteria were essentially clinical, whereas the Poser criteria introduced paraclinical tests to aid diagnostic certainty, and defined clinically definite and laboratory supported MS to assist in defining diagnostic probability. Most recent criteria were outlined by MacDonald et al. in 2001[1] (and usually referred to as the **MacDonald criteria**), and use magnetic resonance imaging (MRI) to help determine further activity on imaging, thereby confirming ongoing inflammation and enabling a diagnosis of MS to be made. These criteria were further revised in 2005[2] (see Tables 4.1–4.3). The MacDonald criteria still rely on the demonstration of areas of inflammation in different parts of the central nervous system at different times, but now permit the use of MRI to define new areas, rather than relying on purely clinical grounds.

Table 4.1 Magnetic resonance imaging criteria for brain abnormality

Three of four of the following:

1. One gadolinium-enhancing lesion or nine T2-hyperintense lesions if there is no gadolinium-enhancing lesion.
2. At least one infratentorial lesion.
3. At least one juxtacortical lesion.
4. At least three periventricular lesions.

Note: A spinal cord lesion can be considered equivalent to a brain infratentorial lesion: an enhancing spinal cord lesion is considered to be equivalent to an enhancing brain lesion, and individual spinal cord lesions can contribute together with individual brain lesions to reach the required number of T2 lesions.

Table 4.2 Magnetic resonance imaging criteria for dissemination of lesions in time

1. There are two ways to show dissemination in time using imaging:
   a. Detection of gadolinium enhancement at least 3 months after the onset of the initial clinical event, if not at the site corresponding to the initial clinical event.
   b. Detection of a new T2 lesion if it appears at any time compared with a reference scan done at least 30 days after the onset of the initial clinical event.

---

1 McDonald WI et al. Recommended diagnostic criteria for multiple sclerosis: guidelines from the international panel on the diagnosis of multiple sclerosis. Ann Neurol 2001; **50**: 121–7.

2 Polman CH et al. Diagnostic criteria for multiple sclerosis: 2005 revisions to the McDonald criteria. Ann Neurol 2005; **58**: 840–6.

Table 4.3 The MacDonald criteria (with 2005 revisions) for making a diagnosis of MS

Clinical presentation	Additional data needed for MS diagnosis
Two or more attacks; objective clinical evidence of 2 or more lesions	None[a]
Two or more attacks; objective clinical evidence of 1 lesion	Dissemination in space, demonstrated by: MRI[b] *or* Two or more MRI-detected lesions consistent with MS plus positive CSF[c] *or* Await further clinical attack implicating a different site
One attack; objective clinical evidence of 2 or more lesions	Dissemination in time, demonstrated by: MRI[d] *or* Second clinical attack
One attack; objective clinical evidence of 1 lesion (mono-symptomatic presentation; clinically isolated syndrome)	Dissemination in space, demonstrated by: MRI[b] *or* Two or more MRI-detected lesions consistent with MS plus positive CSF[c] *and* Dissemination in time, demonstrated by: MRI[d] *or* Second clinical attack
Insidious neurological progression suggestive of MS	1. One year of disease progression (retrospectively or prospectively determined) 2. Plus two of the following: a. Positive brain MRI (nine T2 lesions or four or more T2 lesions with positive VEP) b. Positive spinal cord MRI (two focal T2 lesions) c. Positive CSF[c]

If criteria indicated are fulfilled, the diagnosis is multiple sclerosis (MS); if the criteria are not completely met, the diagnosis is 'possible MS'; if the criteria are fully explored and not met, the diagnosis is 'not MS.'

[a] No additional tests are required; however, if tests [magnetic resonance imaging (MRI), cerebral spinal fluid (CSF)] are undertaken and are *negative*, extreme caution should be taken before making a diagnosis of MS. Alternative diagnoses must be considered. There must be no better explanation for the clinical picture.
[b] MRI demonstration of space dissemination must fulfil the criteria derived from Barkhof et al. and Tintoré et al. (see Table 4.1).
[c] Positive CSF determined by oligoclonal bands detected by established methods (preferably isoelectric focusing) different from any such bands in serum or by a raised IgG index.
[d] MRI demonstration of time dissemination must fulfil the criteria listed in Table 4.2.
[e] Abnormal visual evoked potential of the type seen in MS (delay with well-preserved wave form).

Epidemiology of MS

Prevalence, incidence, and geographical variation

There has been considerable debate over the extent to which genetics or environment play a role in the development of MS and its subsequent disease course: the nature versus nurture controversy. Epidemiological studies of **incidence** (usually quoted as cases/100,000 population/year) and **prevalence** (number of people with MS at any one time in 100,000 population) within specific populations, together with population migration studies, have helped to illuminate some of these issues.

Early studies seemed to demonstrate a **geographical variation** of disease prevalence, in that areas of northern Europe, America, Southern Africa, and Australia had higher levels than parts of central Africa, Asia, and equatorial regions. This led to the concept of a latitudinal gradient, with varying levels even within different parts of the same country such as Australia or the USA. Prevalence maps have been drawn up across the world, with parts of northern Europe and America having levels around 100–150/100,000 population, whereas parts of southern Europe may have levels around 20–50/100,000. Some of the highest levels anywhere in the world have been described in certain areas of Scotland with levels as high as 1 in 500, although most of the UK, northern Europe, and North America will have a level of around 1 in 850. The incidence of MS in areas of high prevalence is around 7/100,000/year.

When interpreting epidemiological data, it remains difficult to separate high prevalence levels due to genetic factors, from possible environmental triggers and from those where migration has occurred (e.g. to parts of Australia from the UK).

Migration studies

Migration studies from areas of low prevalence to areas of high prevalence (such as occurred in migration of West Indians to the UK in the 1950s and 60s), have shown that if people migrated in childhood, then they assumed the higher rate of prevalence of their adopted country, whereas migrating later in life conferred the lower susceptibility of the native West Indies. This led to the concept of environmental exposure occurring before adolescence in genetically predisposed individuals.

Evidence from the Faroe Islands has been used to support the concept that the environmental exposure is in fact an infectious agent. The Faroe Islands are linked administratively with Denmark, an area of high disease prevalence, yet no cases of MS were apparently described in the Faroese population before the Second World War, at which time Allied troops were stationed on these islands. Authors of these studies have been careful in attempting to ensure that lack of evidence prior to the 1940s was not simply due to lack of case ascertainment. There then followed what appear to be a series of epidemics of MS, with peaks of disease incidence every few years. Most cases seemed to be occurring in areas in which troops were stationed, although these were also areas of higher population density. Specific infectious agents have been looked for, but none have been identified as culprits either in the Faroes or anywhere else in the world.

Chapter 6

The natural history of MS

What is natural history?

The natural history of a disease is derived from studies of a population of people with that condition, identified as near as possible to the start of the condition and followed-up longitudinally over as many years as possible, using appropriate measurements. In chronic diseases such as MS these studies can be fraught with difficulties, including adequate case ascertainment (making sure that the investigators have found as many people as possible with MS in the population under study), good long-term follow-up with low rates of dropout (to reduce bias), and choosing the correct measurement instruments. Bias can be introduced by, for example, not taking proper account of mildly affected or severely affected individuals. The introduction of new treatments may also influence the natural history of the condition, a factor relevant in recent years. More broad changes in healthcare may mean that interpreting data derived from cohorts of patients identified 30 years ago may well be different to data derived from patients diagnosed in the twenty-first century.

Knowledge of the natural history of MS is important when counselling people with the condition, although we should always remember that translating from populations to individuals cannot happen easily. Although there are factors that convey good or bad prognosis in general terms, the disease remains fundamentally unpredictable. It is therefore best to approach these issues by stating the facts as honestly and openly as possible:

- It is impossible to predict the prognosis with any degree of certainty in any individual.
- We can learn general facts from studies of large populations of people with MS.
- These facts may influence treatment decisions.

Although there have been many natural history studies, all have used the EDSS as the main clinical measurement, which has many limitations (described in Chapter 9). Perhaps the three main studies that have influenced the literature are the data derived from Ontario, Denmark and Lyons. These and other studies have enabled some important conclusions to be reached which can be used to inform patients and clinical decision-making.

Death from MS

People newly diagnosed with MS can be reassured that rapid fulminant MS leading to death is extremely rare. Overall, there is a slight reduction in survival compared with those people without MS, so that, depending on the age of diagnosis and various other factors, MS may be associated with a reduction of 5–10 years in overall life expectancy.

Disability

The most commonly quoted and useful statistic is that after 15 years of MS, about 50% of people will still be independent in terms of walking, and 50% will be more disabled, requiring use of a stick, wheelchair, or worse. There is now mounting evidence that when people get to the point of requiring persistent help with walking (EDSS 4.0), then they are likely to progress, irrespective of whether they are still having superimposed relapses, or whether they have primary or secondary progressive disease.

Factors predicting outcome

The following factors may be useful in discussing prognosis and treatment options in people with MS. Again, it is important to stress that nothing is absolute, and because this information is derived from population data, it is difficult to translate to the individual.

Factors associated with relatively good outcome:
- Female
- Starting with optic neuritis
- Mainly sensory signs and symptoms
- Little to find on neurological examination
- Low relapse frequency over the first few years
- Lack of problems in coordination and walking
- No evidence of progression
- Low level of lesions on T2 MRI.

Factors associated with relatively worse outcome:
- Male
- Commencing with major balance or walking problems
- Neurological signs of cerebellar and pyramidal disturbance
- High initial relapse frequency (around 5/year)
- Progressive disease
- High level of lesions on T2 MRI.

Chapter 7

Genetics of MS

Twin studies

The classical method for establishing the genetic component to any condition is through twin studies. **Monozygotic** twins are identical and share the same egg, and are therefore identical genetically, so that any differences between them should be accounted for by environmental factors. **Dizygotic** twins occur when two eggs are fertilized simult-aneously, and they are therefore genetically different, but share genes as would siblings within a family. By comparing prevalence rates in these two types of twins, the genetic contribution to any specific condition can be estimated; where twins both have the conditions they are said to be concordant for that condition. There have been many twin studies in MS, and results suggest that monzygotic twin concordance is around 25–30%, whereas dizygotic twin concordance is similar to sibling concordance, around 3–5%. Specific rates can be obtained for the risk of developing MS among family members if there is one affected member of the family (proband). These range from 4.4% for sister, 3.2% (brother), 2% for parents, 0.6% for daughters and 0.6% for sons.

Table 7.1 Risks of developing MS in different populations

1 in 3	Risk to one identical twin when the other twin has MS
1 in 30	Risk to first-degree relative when single family member affected
1 in 500	Risk of developing MS in certain parts of Scotland
1 in 850	Risk of developing MS in most of UK, Northern Europe, and N. America
1 in 2,500	Risk of developing MS in Southern Europe

Genetic associations and linkage

Results from twin studies as well as information about higher incidence of MS in families led to considerable effort being expended in attempting to identify which genes may be associated with either disease susceptibility or disease pattern. Most early studies involved small numbers of patients with results that could not be reproduced. This was largely due to the failure of investigators to make necessary statistical corrections for multiple comparisons, a problem which has affected many areas of genetic research. The only association that seems to have withstood the test of time across different populations is the increased frequency of certain alleles within the **MHC region of chromosome 6**.

To the non-geneticist this area of research can be difficult to follow, not least because the terminology has changed over the four decades since the initial associations with MHC class I HLA-A3 and B7 were first described. It was subsequently found that these alleles are often found tightly linked to MHC class II markers HLA-DR2 and DQw6 (this is known as linkage dysequilibrium). These molecules can be identified using cellular markers on the cell surface (cellular typing allele Dw2), which is the phenotypic expression of specific genes (genotype), namely DRB1*1501, DRB5*0101 (DR15) and DQA1*0102, DQB2*0602 (DQ6). These associations exist for northern European populations, whereas other associations exist for other areas (e.g. Mediterranean association with HLA-DR4).

Associations are frequencies calculated by evaluating the frequency of particular alleles in the MS population compared with a population of normal controls with the same general background. Associations may not be statistically significant if the background levels of these particular genes are high. An alternative way of investigating genes is to look for **linkage** between marker genes and affected/unaffected individuals within families, to see if the disease segregates (is more commonly found in conjunction) with a particular gene or genetic marker. This can be exploited further in more systematic searching of the entire genome, where markers distributed across the genome are used to establish what the likelihood is that none, one, or two alleles are shared at each point. The probability of linkage can be defined as a 'LOD' score (logarithm of the odds) for each marker used (with LOD scores >3 indicating areas of particular interest), which can then be plotted into maps of each chromosome. Further statistical analysis can then determine whether positive LOD scores are likely to encode susceptibility genes.

Despite considerable effort and expenditure, all these studies have not yet identified any specific genetic loci conferring susceptibility or influencing clinical course. Linkage with the known MHC region on chromosome 6 has been confirmed in three separate whole genome studies, but other areas of interest differ according to the population. One reason for the lack of progress in this work may relate to possible disease heterogeneity discussed in the section on pathology (Chapter 2).

Measuring MS

Introduction

Monitoring disease status, evaluating the outcomes of clinical practice, and interpreting the results of research in order to make evidence based judgements about how care should be best delivered, are all skills which are integral to a clinician's role. To undertake this effectively, some understanding of the nature and process of measurement is necessary.

Broadly speaking, measurement of clinical outcomes in MS can be considered at four levels:

1. Physiological parameters of disease, which include lesion load and level of cerebral atrophy.
2. Clinical end-points, which include relapse rate and severity, and hospitalization rates.
3. Aspects of health status, which include levels of activity (disability), participations (handicap), mood and cognitive status.
4. Health related quality of life.

Levels 1 and 2 are often referred to as *physician-based outcomes*; these predominately enhance our understanding of the disease process. In contrast levels 3 and 4 are referred to as *patient-oriented outcomes*, which are so named because they consider outcomes that are important to people with the disease. To provide a comprehensive assessment of the disease process, and its impact on the quantity and quality of an individual's life, it is now generally recognized that all four levels should be considered. When measuring the outcome of health care interventions this is particularly important because research has shown that people with MS and clinicians differ, both in terms of their perceived needs, and as to what constitutes an important and/or successful outcome. If clinicians aim treatments at improving what they judge to be important, without considering the patient's perspective, treatment may be focused on and be evaluated in terms of outcomes that are of little (or no) value to the person with MS.

Deciding what to measure

There are a number of important issues that require careful consideration prior to undertaking any evaluation in order to ensure that relevant and meaningful aspects are measured in a timely and appropriate manner. These include:

- *Understanding the main purpose of the evaluation.* There are many different reasons as to why you might wish to undertake an evaluation. For instance, it may be that you wish to monitor disease or health status, or to evaluate the outcomes of routine clinical practice, or to determine effectiveness of an intervention by undertaking a clinical trial. The purpose of the evaluation will directly influence what you will measure and how you will undertake the measurement process.
- *Understanding the characteristics of the sample* on whom you are carrrying out the measurement. This may include, for instance, the level of severity of the key aspects you are measuring (such as disease severity, level of functional independence, or degree of difficulties with mobility).
- *Understanding the aim of the intervention*, if you are evaluating treatment effectiveness. This requires an understanding both in terms of what the intervention involves and what you are trying to change.
- *Understanding what can be expected to change* as a result of an intervention, the likely size of that change, and when it is most likely to occur. There is little point measuring aspects that you do not think will change with intervention, nor in using a measurement instrument that is unlikely to detect the size of changes that will typically occur.

The World Health Organization's classification system *The International Classification of Functioning Disability and Health* is a useful framework for deciding which aspects may be relevant to measure. It provides a logical continuum for the measurement of disease, which includes measurement of the underlying disease processes (pathology), which results in symptoms and signs (impairment) which can lead to restriction in performing tasks (limitation in activities) and subsequently socio-economic limitations (restriction in participations). This classification system is probably the most widely used framework for measuring disease status and health outcomes, and is discussed in more detail in Chapter 20.

Commonly measured outcomes

Measures of disease activity

Magnetic resonance imaging (MRI) techniques are commonly used to monitor disease activity in clinical trials of MS, since they are now generally acknowledged to highlight the evolving pathology of the disease. For instance, studies have shown good correlation between: lesions seen on MRI and lesions seen on pathology; gadolinium enhancement and inflammatory lesions on biopsy; and unenhanced T1 black holes with axonal loss. In contrast however there is much poorer correlation between MRI lesion load and clinical measures; with only some lesions detected by MRI being reflected by clinical changes. For example studies of T2-weighted and standard dose gadolinium enhanced T1-weighted MRI brain scans of patients in early relapsing remitting MS, have revealed about ten active lesions (i.e. new and/or enhancing) for every clinical relapse. As a consequence, a combination of both MRI and clinical measures are typically used to monitor the impact of MS, and the effectiveness of interventions (Table 8.1). Further information on uses of MRI is found in Chapter 13.

Measures of impairment

Impairment scales are largely based on clinical examination, which may be undertaken by different members of the multi-disciplinary team. They include a diverse range of measures to encompass the wide range of impairments seen in MS. For example, the Expanded Disability Status Scale (EDSS) and its related Functional Systems Scale (FSS) was designed to measure neurological status based on neurological examination; the Ashworth Scale to measure spasticity; and the Medical Research Council Scale to measure muscle strength. Importantly the severity of impairment may not always relate to the functional difficulties or the quality of life experienced by people with MS, and hence in order to gain a fuller picture of the impact of the disease on individuals, it is recommended that measures of impairment should be undertaken in conjunction with clinical rating scales of aspects of health status.

Measures of health status and health-related quality of life

People with MS generally have a normal life expectancy, and so most live with some degree of disability for a prolonged period of time, which invariably has wide ranging impacts on the individual. Clinical rating scales are available to enable standardized measurement of many different aspects of health status which include: activity levels (disability); limitation in participations (handicap); and health-related quality of life. These scales enable classification of individuals according to the degree of difficulties experienced in each of these areas, as well as allowing changes to be detected over time, either as a consequence of intervention, or the natural course of the disease.

Broadly speaking, health status measures can be divided into two groups: generic or disease specific measures. Generic measures are those that are designed to be broadly applicable across different types and severity of disease, medical interventions, and demographic and cultural

Table 8.1 Typical outcomes measured in MS clinical trials

Acute clinical activity	
1. Clinical measures	• Number of relapses • Severity of relapses • Hospitalizations for relapses
2. MRI measures	• New lesions—number and duration • Enlarging lesions—number and duration • Stable lesions • Enhancing lesions—number and area
Chronic clinical activity	
1. Clinical measures	• Impairment scales • Scales of activity (disability) • Ambulation scales
2. MRI measures	• Measures of the extent of disease T1 unenhanced, T2 (lesion load) • Measures of atrophy

groups so as to permit comparisons across studies. The Medical Outcome Study Short Form-36 (SF-36) is a well-known example of a generic measure of health status. In contrast disease-specific measures are designed to reflect clinically relevant issues for a specific disease. Recently, many disease-specific measures for MS have been developed for use in evaluating MS and treatment effectiveness. A brief description of some of these is provided in the following section. Unfortunately none of the scales completely satisfy the clinical (feasibility, acceptability) and scientific requirements of outcome measures (reliability, validity, and responsiveness—see below), although each have some desirable properties. Perhaps as a consequence, none has been universally accepted for use, which has led to difficulties in interpreting and comparing the effectiveness of interventions.

Important clinical and psychometric considerations when choosing a measurement instrument

For most clinicians in routine clinical practice, measurement is undertaken through the use of standardized assessment scales. When choosing which scale to use, it is essential to remember that the value of any measurement instrument depends on its clinical usefulness and scientific robustness. Consideration of these factors is important both within the context of assessing individuals within routine clinical practice, or populations within clinical trials.

Clinical usefulness is concerned with aspects of the measure that concern implementation into clinical practice. A scale that is clinically useful should be practical to administer and cost efficient. It should also be acceptable to the individual being assessed and to the professional using it.

Scientific robustness is concerned with the scientific rigor of the instrument in terms of three basic psychometric properties:

- **Reliability**: considers whether a measure is consistent, produces accurate results, is stable over time, and is reproducible. It addresses the internal consistency of the scale items (in multidimensional scales) and the reproducibility of the scores when the instrument is applied by the same (intra-) or a different (inter-) rater, or by the same patient (test–retest) in the case of self-rating measures. The reliability of a measure has clear practical implications since it determines important issues such as the number of raters that should assess the patient in order to optimize reliability; the level of training required by raters; and the need to use protocols or manuals.

- **Validity**: considers whether the instrument measures the concept which is intended to be measured. It is usually established by expert opinion (face and content validity), and by demonstrating a high correlation between the instrument and a gold standard (criterion validity). In the absence of a gold standard, validity is established by assessing the degree to which the scale correlates with other existing measures of related (convergent construct validity) or unrelated constructs (discriminant construct validity), and with hypothesis testing, or by testing its ability to differentiate between patient groups known to differ in the concept being measured (group differences).
  Information about the validity of a measure can generally be found within the developer's manual (if one exists), and/or within journal articles. Increasingly, information is also being made available on the internet by the developers.

- **Responsiveness**: assesses the ability of the scale to detect clinically meaningful change. Knowledge about the responsiveness of an instrument is crucial to interpret the results it generates in an informed manner. A scale that has poor responsiveness, for instance, may not detect clinically significant change that has occurred, thereby potentially misleading the interpretation of results by suggesting that the intervention was not effective.

- **Appropriateness** is a term that has been used to describe the score distribution of a scale. When used in a large sample, the scores should have a near normal distribution with no 'floor' or 'ceiling' effects. This allows discrimination between patients with varying degrees of disease severity.

It is important to remember that reliability, validity and reponsiveness are all sample dependent. Hence it is essential to find out whether these properties have been established in different samples (for example different levels of functional ability; or severity of symptoms), and within different settings. Furthermore these properties cannot be established within a single study; and it is important to critically review the literature to determine how extensively the measure has been evaluated. This enables the results to be interpeted in the light of both the strengths and limitations of the measure.

Chapter 9

Frequently used assessment scales

Introduction

A brief description of some of the assessment scales which have been more commonly used within routine MS clinical practice and clinical trials follows. This list is clearly not exhaustive. Furthermore a health warning is given about the information provided; studies evaluating the clinical and psychometric properties of these scales are continually ongoing and as a consequence the information about them becomes quickly out-of-date. This section therefore simply attempts to provide a brief summary of the knowledge gained thus far. Before choosing any of these measures for use it is recommended that you undertake a more thorough review of the literature to gain detailed information about the overall strengths and limitations of the measure in relation to the sample and the setting in which you are intending to use it. There are a number of books that provide a general overview of measures, which can help to direct and focus your search. The detective work undertaken in selecting the most appropriate measure is well worth the time and effort expended, since it will markedly impact on the credibility of the results generated.[1,2]

1 Bowling A. *Measuring Health: a review of quality of life measurement scales.* Open University Press, Buckingham 2005.
2 Finch E, Brooks D, Stratford PW *et al.* *Physical Rehabilitation Outcome Measures: a guide to enhanced decision making.* BC Decker Inc, Ontario 2002.

The Expanded Disability Status Scale (EDSS) and Functional Systems Scales (FSS)

Description

The EDSS is the best known and the most widely used scale in clinical trials of MS. Based on the results of the neurological examination the EDSS is a 20-step ordinal scale, which ranges from 0 (normal neurological status) to 10 (death due to MS complications). It predominately evaluates impairment in the early levels (0–3.5), mobility in the middle range (4.0–7.5) and upper limb (8.0–8.5) and bulbar function in the late stages (9.0–9.5), although the total score is biased towards ambulation (Table 9.1). EDSS steps 1.0 to 4.5 refer to people who are fully ambulatory, while steps 5.0 to 9.5 are essentially defined by level of difficulty with ambulation. The eight FSS allow the neurologist to assign a score to each of the following systems: pyramidal, cerebellar, brainstem, sensory, bowel and bladder, visual, mood/cognition, and other. Each of the FSS and the EDSS are single-item scales and there is no composite or summed score.

Administration time and method

The FSS and EDSS are administered in person by a trained examiner, most often a neurologist. Administration time varies depending upon the condition of the patient and the skill of the examiner with the neurological examination required, so that the assessment can take anywhere between 15 and 30 minutes.

Psychometric properties

Both test–retest and inter-rater reliability have varied considerably from study to study with some studies finding high values and other studies unacceptably low values. Responsiveness has been demonstrated to be poor relative to other measures of impairment and disability, and to patient and clinician assessment of change.

Developer's reference:

Kurtzke JF. Rating neurologic impairment in multiple sclerosis: an expanded disability status scale (EDSS). *Neurology* 1983; **33** (11): 1444–52.

Relevant website:

Downloadable pdf form for the FSS and EDSS: *http://www.nationalmssociety.org/MUCS_FSS.asp*

Table 9.1 Expanded Disability Status Scale

0.0	Normal neurological examination
1.0	No disability, minimal signs in one FS
1.5	No disability, minimal signs in more than one FS
2.0	Minimal disability in one FS
2.5	Mild disability in one FS or minimal disability in two FS
3.0	Moderate disability in one FS, or mild disability in three or four FS. Fully ambulatory
3.5	Fully ambulatory but with moderate disability in one FS and more than minimal disability in several others
4.0	Fully ambulatory without aid, self-sufficient, up and about some 12 hours a day despite relatively severe disability; able to walk without aid or rest for 500 metres
4.5	Fully ambulatory without aid, up and about much of the day, able to work a full day, may otherwise have some limitation of full activity or require minimal assistance; characterized by relatively severe disability; able to walk without aid or rest for 300 metres
5.0	Ambulatory without aid or rest for about 200 metres; disability severe enough to impair full daily activities (work a full day without special provisions)
5.5	Ambulatory without aid or rest for about 100 metres; disability severe enough to preclude full daily activities
6.0	Intermittent or unilateral constant assistance (cane, crutch, brace) required to walk about 100 metres with or without resting
6.5	Constant bilateral assistance (canes, crutches, braces) required to walk about 20 metres without resting
7.0	Unable to walk beyond approximately five metres even with aid, essentially restricted to wheelchair; wheels self in standard wheelchair and transfers alone; up and about in wheelchair some 12 hours a day
7.5	Unable to take more than a few steps; restricted to wheelchair; may need aid in transfer; wheels self but cannot carry on in standard wheelchair a full day; may require motorized wheelchair
8.0	Essentially restricted to bed or chair or perambulated in wheelchair, but may be out of bed itself much of the day; retains many self-care functions; generally has effective use of arms
8.5	Essentially restricted to bed much of day; has some effective use of arms; retains some self care functions
9.0	Confined to bed; can still communicate and eat
9.5	Totally helpless bed patient; unable to communicate effectively or eat/swallow
10.0	Death due to MS

Multiple Sclerosis Functional Composite (MSFC)

Description

The MSFC is a three-part, standardized, quantitative assessment instrument designed for use in clinical trials of MS (Table 9.2). The three measures making up the MSFC evaluate leg function/ambulation (timed 25 foot walk), upper limb function (nine-hole peg test), and cognitive function (Paced Auditory Serial Addition Test—PASAT). The MSFC was developed by a special task force on clinical outcomes assessment who felt that existing measures (particularly the EDSS) failed to address important clinical dimensions, such as cognition, and demonstrated poor responsiveness to clinically meaningful change.

Administration time and method

The MSFC is administered in person by a trained examiner, who may not necessarily be a neurologist. The total time for administration of all three measures varies depending upon the ability of the patient, but is typically in the region of 20–30 minutes. Patients often find the PASAT intimidating and compliance can be a problem.

Scoring

The MSFC can produce scores for each of its three individual measures as well as a composite score. In addition, there are a variety of ways to calculate scores depending on the nature of the study and the sample. These are described in the administration and scoring manual (accessible at *http://www.nationalmssociety.org/MUCS_MSFC.asp*).

Psychometric properties

All three measures making up the MSFC have been shown to have good inter-rater and test-retest reliability. In addition, there is reasonable evidence for their validity and responsiveness in people with MS. Performance on the MSFC is however sensitive to practice effects, with patients often displaying poorer performance when first tested due to lack of familiarity with the tasks. It is therefore recommended that three or four administrations be given prior to a baseline assessment to optimize accuracy of assessments of change over time.

Developer's reference:

Cutter GR, Baier ML, Rudick RA *et al.* Development of a multiple sclerosis functional composite as a clinical trial outcome measure. *Brain* 1999; **122** (5): 871–82

Relevant websites:

Downloadable administration and scoring manual:
http://www.nationalmssociety.org/MUCS_MSFC.asp

Table 9.2 Multiple Sclerosis Functional Composite (MSFC)

25 foot timed walk (The first component administered).	• Time taken to walk 25 foot, as quickly and safely as possible. • The test is undertaken twice, and an average determined.
Nine-hole peg test (The second component administered).	• Time taken to pick up 9 pegs one at a time as quickly as possible, put them in 9 holes, and, once they are in the holes, remove them again as quickly as possible one at a time, replacing them into a shallow container. • Both the dominant and non-dominant hands are tested twice; the score is the average of the 4 trials.
The PASAT (The third component administered).	This measures cognitive function by assessing auditory information processing speed and flexibility, as well as calculation ability. An audiocassette tape presents single digits every 3 seconds and the patient must add each new digit to the one immediately prior to it.

Guy's Neurological Disability Scale (renamed the UK Neurological Disability Scale)

Description

The Guy's Neurological Disability Scale (GNDS) was designed as a clinical disability scale capable of embracing the whole range of disabilities encountered in MS. It has 12 separate categories including cognition, mood, vision, speech, swallowing, upper limb function, lower limb function, bladder function, bowel function, sexual function, fatigue, and 'others'. A sample item from the scale (mood) is detailed in Table 9.3.

Administration time and method

This scale can be administered by self report, by phone or face to face interview, or via a postal questionnaire. The interview can be undertaken by neurologists and non-neurologists. It takes approximately 10 minutes to administer.

Scoring

The level of disability is graded in each of the 12 categories (Table 9.4). A total score is also calculated by summing the 12 separate sub-scores, giving a sum score ranging between zero (no disability) and 60 (maximum disability).

Psychometric qualities

The GNDS has been found to be acceptable to neurologists and patients. Its reliability, validity and responsiveness has been demonstrated as a measure of disability in both hospital and community settings, and with each of the different methods of administration.

Table 9.3 Sample interview item from the Guy's (now UK) Neurological Disability Scale

Instructions

This scale is designed to assess disability in patients with MS. It has 12 separate categories each with an interview and scoring section. The total GNDS score is the sum of the 12 separate scores. The questions are directed to assess the disability in the previous one month.

Question 2. Mood disability

A. Interview:

Have you been feeling anxious, irritable, depressed or had any mood swings during the last month?

Yes ☐   No ☐

Are you taking any medication for such problem?

Yes ☐   No ☐

If the answer to the first question is 'yes':

Has the problem affected your ability to do *any* of your usual daily activities such as work, housework, or normal social activity with family and friends?

Yes ☐   No ☐

If 'yes'

Has this problem been severe enough to prevent you from doing *all* your usual activities?

Yes ☐   No ☐

Have you been admitted to hospital for treatment of your mood problem during the last month?

Yes ☐   No ☐

Table 9.4 Severity grades for Guy's (now UK) Neurological Disability Scale

Grade	Level of disability
0	Normal status
1	Symptoms causing no disability
2	Mild disability—not requiring help from others
3	Moderate disability—requiring help from others
4	Severe disability—almost total loss of function
5	Total loss of function—maximum help required

Developer's reference:

Sharrack B, Hughes RAC. The Guy's Neurological Disability Scale (GNDS): a new disability measure for multiple sclerosis. *Multiple Sclerosis* 1999; **5** (4): 223–33. N.B. This article appendixes a full version of the rating scale, together with scoring procedure.

The Barthel Index (BI)

Description

The BI measures functional independence in personal care and mobility, principally in terms of physical aspects of disability. It is performance-based, that is, it records what a patient does, not what a patient could do. The main aim of this measure is to establish degree of independence from any help, physical or verbal, however minor and for whatever reason.

Administration time and method

Scoring takes approximately 20 minutes if performance is observed, or 5 minutes if information is obtained by self-report.

Scoring

This is a 10 item ordinal scale, which gives a score from 0–20 (Table 9.5).

Psychometric properties

The BI has been validated for use in people with a wide range of conditions, including MS, and may be performed in a rehabilitation unit, clinic or community settings. Reliability and validity has shown to be good with different methods of administration (including postal administration) and across different settings. The BI has shown to be responsive to changes in function in association with interventions such as multi-disciplinary rehabilitation in people with MS.

General comments

A perfect score does not mean that the person is able to live alone or to perform domestic activities of daily living such as cooking or cleaning. Generally speaking, a score of 14 indicates some disability, usually compatible with the level of support found in a residential home, and a score of 10 compatible with discharge home provided there is maximum support and a carer in attendance.

Developer's reference:

Mahoney FI, Barthel D. Functional evaluation: the Barthel Index. *Maryland State Medical Journal* 1965; **14**: 56–61.

Relevant website:

Downloadable form and calculator: *http://info.med.yale.edu/neurol/residency/barthel.html*

Table 9.5 The Barthel Index (observed)

Activity	Criterion	Score
Feeding	Unable	0
	Needs help cutting, spreading butter, etc.	1
	Independent	2
Using bath or shower	Needs help	0
	Independent	1
Grooming (teeth, hair, shaving, washing)	Needs help	0
	Independent	1
Dressing	Unable, dependent	0
	Needs help but can do about half unaided	1
	Independent (including buttons, zips, laces)	2
Bowel continence	Incontinent: >once per week (or needs to be given enemas)	0
	Occasional accident: <once per week	1
	Continent	2
Bladder continence	Incontinent: ≥once a day, or catheterized and unable to manage alone	0
	Occasional accident: wet <once per day	1
	Continent	2
Toilet use	Unable or fully dependent	0
	Needs some help, but does some things alone	1
	Independent (including getting on and off toilet, dressing, wiping)	2
Transfers (bed to chair and back)	Unable, no sitting balance, cannot stand	0
	Major help (can sit, needs one or two people)	1
	Minor help (verbal or physical of one)	2
	Independent	3
Walking (on level surfaces, using any aid)	Immobile	0
	Wheelchair independent, including corners	1
	Walks with help of one person (verbal or physical)	2
	Independent (may use any aid) >10 metres	3
Stairs	Unable	0
	Needs help (verbal, physical, carrying aid)	1
	Independent	2
Available score range		0–20

The Functional Independence Measure (FIM)

Description

The FIM is a generic measure that rates the level of assistance required to perform basic activities of daily living across a range of motor and cognitive functions (Table 9.6). In doing so it provides an estimate of burden of care and cost of disability.

Administration time and method

Scores are based on observation, although telephone and face-to-face interviews have also been used as a method of administration. If scoring is based on clinical observation, the time taken to administer is in the region of 45 minutes. Scoring based on interview takes approximately 15 minutes. Scoring can be undertaken by any discipline but the evaluator must be trained.

Scoring

The domains covered in the FIM are: self care, sphincter control, transfers, locomotion, communication, and social cognition. Eighteen items (13 motor, 5 cognition) are rated on a seven level ordinal scale, with scores ranging between 18 (total dependence) and 126 (highest level of independence).

Psychometric properties

The FIM has undergone extensive psychometric testing and has been shown to be reliable, valid and responsive in a range of conditions (including MS); across a range of different settings, and with different methods of administration. While reliability of summed sub-scale scores has been demonstrated to be good, inter- and intra-rater reliabilities have proven variable with individual item scores. The FIM has shown to be responsive to change in association with interventions such as physiotherapy and multi-disciplinary rehabilitation in MS.

Table 9.6 The Functional Independence Measure

Sub-scale items	Criterion
Motor items	*Score 1 (Total assistance):*
Eating	the subject expends less than 25% of the effort to perform an activity.
Grooming	
Bathing	*Score 2 (Maximal assistance):*
Dressing: upper body	the patient expends 25–49% of the effort to perform an activity.
Dressing: lower body	
Toileting	*Score 3 (Moderate assistance):*
Bladder management	the subject requires more help than touching or expends half or more (but less than 75%) of the effort to perform an activity.
Bowel management	
Transfers: bed, chair, wheelchair	
Transfers: toilet	*Score 4 (Minimal contact assistance):*
Transfers: bath or shower	the subject requires no more help than touching and expends 75% or more of the effort to perform the activity.
Locomotion: walk, wheelchair	
Stairs	
Cognitive items	*Score 5 (Supervision or set-up):*
Comprehension	this refers to help such as standby or distant supervision, cueing or coaxing without physical contact, set up of needed items, or application of orthoses.
Expression	
Social interaction	
Problem solving	*Score 6 (Modified independence):*
Memory	the activity requires an assistive device, the activity takes more than reasonable time, or there are safety (risk) considerations.
	Score 7 (Complete independence):
	all of the tasks described as making up the activity are performed safely, without modification, assistive devices, or aids, and within a reasonable amount of time.

Developer's reference:

Granger CV, Cotter AS, Hamilton BB et al. Functional assessment scales: A study of persons with multiple sclerosis. *Archives Physical Medicine and Rehabilitation* 1990; **71**: 870–5.

Relevant website:

http://www.udsmr.org

The 12-item Multiple Sclerosis Walking Scale (MSWS-12)

Description

The MSWS-12 is a questionnaire that asks the patient to rate the degree of limitation in walking, due to MS, experienced in the prior 2 weeks (Table 9.7). The 12 items were generated from patient interviews, expert opinion, and literature review.

Administration time and methods

The questionnaire is self-completed by the patient. On average this takes approximately 5 minutes.

Scoring

Individual item responses in the MSWS-12 are summed to generate a total score and this value is then transformed to a scale with a range of 0–100. Higher scores reflect a greater limitation on walking abilities related to MS.

Psychometric properties

The scale has demonstrated to have good validity and test-retest reliability in people with MS, used in different settings (community and hospital). The MSWS-12 has been found to be more responsive in detecting change in mobility than a range of other health status measures, such as the Functional Assessment of MS mobility scale, Short Form-36 physical functioning scale, EDSS and the timed walk test.

Table 9.7 The Multiple Sclerosis Walking Scale

In the past two weeks, how much has your MS ...

1. Limited your ability to walk?
2. Limited your ability to run?
3. Limited your ability to climb up and down stairs?
4. Made standing when doing things more difficult?
5. Limited your balance when standing or walking?
6. Limited how far you are able to walk?
7. Increased the effort needed for you to walk?
8. Made it necessary for you to use support when walking indoors (e.g. holding on to furniture, using a stick, etc)?
9. Made it necessary for you to use support when walking outdoors (e.g. using a stick, a frame, etc)?
10. Slowed down your walking?
11. Affected how smoothly you walk?
12. Made you concentrate on your walking?

Scoring

Each item is scored on a scale of scale of one to five where: not at all = 1; a little = 2; moderately = 3; quite a bit = 4; extremely = 5

Developer's reference:
Hobart JC, Riazi A, Lamping DL. *et al.* Measuring the impact of MS on walking ability: the 12-item MS walking scale (MSWS-12). *Neurology* 2003; **60**: 31–6.
Relevant website with downloadable form and scoring procedure: *www.pms.ac.uk/cnrg*.

The Modified Fatigue Impact Scale (MFIS)

Description

The MFIS is a modified form of the Fatigue Impact Scale which is based on items derived from interviews with MS patients concerning how fatigue impacts their lives. This 21 item scale assesses the effects of fatigue in terms of physical, cognitive, and psychosocial functioning (Table 9.8). A shorter 5-item version is also available.

Administration time and method

This structured, self-report questionnaire takes approximately 10 minutes to complete for the full-length version and 2–3 minutes for the abbreviated version. Interview administration can be undertaken in patients with visual or upper extremity impairments.

Scoring

Subjects rate their fatigue using a 5 point scale from 0 (no problem, fatigue *never* affects the activity) to 4 (extreme problem, fatigue *almost always* affects the activity). The total score for the MFIS is the sum of the scores for the 21 items, with a potential range of 0 to 84. Individual subscale scores for *physical, cognitive*, and *psychosocial functioning* can also be generated by calculating the sum of specific sets of items. Higher scores indicate a greater impact of fatigue on the person's activities.

Psychometric properties

The reliability and validity of this scale has been determined in a number of studies, which have included hospitalized and community based patients. It has demonstrated to be responsive to changes following interventions such as medications for fatigue and inpatient rehabilitation. The authors report that the availability of the 3 subscales, physical, cognitive, and psychosocial functioning, can be useful to investigators interested in testing hypotheses concerning these different areas of function. It has been noted, however, that the 3 subscales tend to correlate highly with one another, which limits their usefulness to some extent.

Table 9.8 Modified Fatigue Impact Scale

Because of my fatigue during the past 4 weeks ...

1. I have been less alert
2. I have had difficulty paying attention for long periods of time
3. I have been unable to think clearly
4. I have been clumsy and uncoordinated
5. I have been forgetful
6. I have had to pace myself in my physical activities
7. I have been less motivated to do anything that requires physical effort
8. I have been less motivated to participate in social activities
9. I have been limited in my ability to do things away from home
10. I have trouble maintaining physical effort for long periods
11. I have had difficulty making decisions
12. I have been less motivated to do anything that requires thinking
13. My muscles have felt weak
14. I have been physically uncomfortable
15. I have had trouble finishing tasks that require thinking
16. I have had difficulty organizing my thoughts when doing things at home or at work
17. I have been less able to complete tasks that require physical effort
18. My thinking has been slowed down
19. I have had trouble concentrating
20. I have limited my physical activities
21. I have needed to rest more often or for longer periods.

Scoring:

Each item is scored on a scale of scale of 0 to 4 where: never = 0; rarely = 1; sometimes = 2; often = 3; almost always = 4

Developer's reference:

Fisk JD, Ritvo PG, Ross L et al. Measuring the functional impact of fatigue: initial validation of the fatigue impact scale. *Clinical Infectious Diseases* 1994; **18** (Suppl1): S79–83.

Relevant website:

The MFIS is part of the MS Quality of Life Inventory, which can be downloaded, together with scoring instructions, from:

http://www.nationalmssociety.org/pdf/research/MSQLI_Manual_and_Forms.pdf

Fatigue Severity Scale (FSS)

Description

The FSS is a multidimensional assessment scale for evaluating fatigue in MS and other conditions. It was designed to assist clinicians in recognizing and diagnosing fatigue and to differentiate fatigue from clinical depression, since both share some of the same symptoms. The questionnaire consists of 9 statements that attempt to explore severity of fatigue symptoms as they relate to daily activities.

Administration time and method

This structured self-report questionnaire takes approximately 5 minutes to complete and score. The person is asked to read each statement and circle a number from 1 to 7, depending on how appropriate they feel the statement applies to them over the preceding week (Table 9.9).

Scoring

Scoring is based on a scale ranging from 1 to 7 where 1 means the person strongly disagrees with the statement and 7 means they strongly agree with the statement. The score is calculated by averaging the responses to the question (total of all responses divided by 9). The possible score range is 1 to 7. The developers suggest that people with depression alone score about 4.5, whereas people with fatigue related to MS average about 6.5.

Psychometric properties

Studies evaluating the psychometric properties are relatively limited. However those undertaken show the scale to be internally consistent, to correlate moderately well with a single item visual analogue scale of fatigue intensity, to clearly differentiate controls from patients, and to detect clinical changes in fatigue over time in people with MS. A ceiling effect may limit its utility to assess severe fatigue-related disability.

Table 9.9 The Fatigue Severity Scale

During the past week, I have found that:

1. My motivation is lower when I am fatigued.

2. Exercise brings on my fatigue.

3. I am easily fatigued.

4. Fatigue interferes with my physical functioning.

5. Fatigue causes frequent problems for me.

6. My fatigue prevents sustained physical functioning.

7. Fatigue interferes with carrying out certain duties and responsibilities.

8. Fatigue is among my three most disabling symptoms.

9. Fatigue interferes with my work, family, or social life.

Scoring:

Each item is scored on a scale of 1 to 7 where a lower score indicates low agreement with the statement, and a high score indicates high agreement

Developer's reference:

Krupp LB et *al.* The Fatigue Severity Scale: application to patients with multiple sclerosis and systemic lupus erythematosis. *Archives of Neurology* 1989; **46**: 1121–23.

Relevant website:

A printable version of the scale with scoring instructions is available at:

http://www.healthywomen.org/healthtopics/sleepdisorders/fatigueseverityscalefss

Multiple Sclerosis Quality of Life-54 Instrument (MSQOL-54)

Description

The MSQOL-54 is a multidimensional health-related quality of life measure which combines both generic and MS-specific items into a single instrument. It contains 36 items from the Short-Form 36 (SF-36) generic health related quality of life scale, plus 18 MS-specific items (addressing issues such as fatigue, cognitive impairment, and sexual function).

Scoring

There is no single overall score for this 54-item instrument. Two summary scores—*physical health* and *mental health*—can be derived from a weighted combination of scale scores. In addition the scale generates 12 subscales and two additional single-item measures (Table 9.10).

Administration time and method

This is a structured, self-report questionnaire that the patient can generally complete with little or no assistance. It may also be administered by an interviewer. Administration time is approximately 10–20 minutes.

Psychometric qualities

Psychometric evaluation of this 54-item scale is relatively limited. Studies by the developers have demonstrated high internal consistency and test-retest reliability, and there is some evidence supporting its discriminant validity across different levels of disability. Other studies, however, have raised concerns about its validity and responsiveness, demonstrating marked floor and ceiling effects and relatively poor responsiveness for a number of the dimensions.

General comments

The MSQOL-54 includes as its core 36 items from one of the most widely used quality of life measures, the SF-36, which has had extensive psychometric testing. Availability of population-based normative data for the SF-36 portion of the MSQOL-54 makes this component of the instrument useful for comparative purposes.

Table 9.10 The Multiple Sclerosis Quality of Life-54 Instrument

Subscale items

Physical subscales:

Physical function (10 items)

Role limitations—physical (4 items)

Pain (3 items)

Energy (5 items)

Sexual function (4 items)

Mental health subscales:

Role limitations—emotional (3 items)

Emotional well-being (5 items)

Health perceptions (5 items)

Social function (3 items)

Cognitive function (4 items)

Overall quality of life (2 items)

Health distress (4 items)

Single item measures:

Change in health

Satisfaction with sexual function

Scoring

- Physical health composite summary
- Mental health composite summary

Derived from a weighted combination of subscale scores

Developer's reference:

Vickrey BG, Hays RD, Harooni R, *et al.* A health-related quality of life measure for multiple sclerosis. *Quality of Life Research* 1995; **4**: 187–206.

Relevant website:

Downloadable pdf form and scoring instructions (with formulae)

http://www.nationalmssociety.org/MUCS_MSQOL-54.asp

Multiple Sclerosis Impact Scale (MSIS-29)

Description

This MS-specific rating scale measures the physical and psychological impact of MS from the patient's perspective. Its 29 items were generated from patient interviews, expert opinion and literature review (Table 9.11). The developer's intention was to develop a MS-specific outcome measure which combines the patient perspective with a rigorous scientific approach.

Administration time and method

This is a self-report questionnaire which takes approximately 5–10 minutes to complete.

Scoring

Individual item responses in the MSIS-29 are summed to generate a total score with a range of 29–145. The lower the score, the less the perceived impact of the condition on aspects of everyday life.

Psychometric properties

Extensive testing of this scale has been undertaken, demonstrating it to have high internal consistency and test–retest reliability and good validity. Responsiveness has been demonstrated in both hospital and community settings, with different interventions including steroid therapy and rehabilitation, and across the broad spectrum of disease severity.

Table 9.11 The Multiple Sclerosis Impact Scale

In the past 2 weeks, how much has your MS limited your ability to ...

1. Do physically demanding tasks?
2. Grip things tightly (e.g. turning on taps)?
3. Carry things?

In the past 2 weeks, how much have you been bothered by ...

4. Problems with your balance?
5. Difficulties moving about indoors?
6. Being clumsy?
7. Stiffness?
8. Heavy arms and/or legs?
9. Tremor of your arms or legs?
10. Spasms in your limbs?
11. Your body not doing what you want it to do?
12. Having to depend on others to do things for you?
13. Limitations in your social and leisure activities at home?
14. Being stuck at home more than you would like to be?
15. Difficulties using your hands in everyday tasks?
16. Having to cut down the amount of time you spent on work or other daily activities?
17. Problems using transport (e.g. car, bus, train, taxi, etc.)?
18. Taking longer to do things?
19. Difficulty doing things spontaneously (e.g. going out on the spur of the moment)?
20. Needing to go to the toilet urgently?
21. Feeling unwell?
22. Problems sleeping?
23. Feeling mentally fatigued?
24. Worries related to your MS?
25. Feeling anxious or tense?
26. Feeling irritable, impatient, or short tempered?
27. Problems concentrating?
28. Lack of confidence?
29. Feeling depressed?

Scoring:

Each item is scored on a scale of 1 to 5 where:
not at all = 1; a little = 2; moderately = 3; quite a bit = 4; extremely = 5

Developer's reference:

Hobart JC, Lamping DL, Fitzpatrick R, et al. The Multiple Sclerosis Impact Scale (MSIS-29): a new patient-based outcome measure. *Brain* 2001; **124**: 962–73. N.B. This article appendixes a full version of the rating scale.

Relevant website: *www.pms.ac.uk/cnrg*

Chapter 10

How to determine whether treatments are effective

Evidence-based medicine and clinical trials

We are all rightly encouraged to practice evidence-based medicine. That is to say, treatment decisions should be based on a thorough evaluation of the risks and benefits of any treatment, preferably after due consideration of well designed and conducted clinical trials. Because MS is so unpredictable, and treatment options have historically been poor, there is a great tendency for individual patients or doctors to latch onto the latest treatment fad. Before long, such treatments may become used routinely, usually on the basis of anecdote and word of mouth. This is not a good way of basing treatment decisions, and it is important that everyone associated with treating a chronic disease such as MS is aware of the pitfalls in this area.

It is sometimes worth providing people with an example of anecdote, such as the possibility that apples may cure MS. If someone ate a particular type of apple and from that point onwards they had no further relapses, they might suggest that apples are the cure for MS. A more realistic explanation may be that this pattern of disease course would have happened despite the apple, and such effects were simply due to chance. To test the theory, we would need to choose two large groups of people with MS in order to get round the random variation between people, and then randomly allocate treatments to each group, such as apples or pears, or apples against no apples. The randomization process gets round bias that might otherwise make particular doctors prescribe specific treatments to people with better or worse prognosis. If the doctor gave apples to everyone with very mild disease, and no treatment to everyone with more severe disease, the results would favour apples as a treatment, as people in the no treatment group would do worse anyway.

In randomized clinical trials, we usually try to avoid further bias by masking treatment allocation to both patients and doctors (so-called double blind trials). This would be difficult in the case of apples, as they are readily recognizable, but certain drugs may also cause unmasking by their side effects, which could suggest to the participant in the clinical trial which treatment they are receiving. That knowledge may bias their performance or outcome measurement. Ideally, treatment trials compare active treatment to placebo treatment that looks, smells, tastes and feels, the same.

How good is any clinical trial?

In evaluating clinical trials it is worth considering a few important questions:

- Is the main outcome measure appropriate—does it measure what we think it measures (validity), and is it responsive enough to detect change (responsiveness)? Evidence emerging from a variety of sources reinforces the variability in the most commonly used scale to measure MS (the EDSS). Many clinical trials have used EDSS progression of 0.5–1.5 points (depending on where someone starts on the scale at the beginning of the trial) at 2 consecutive points separated by only 3 months. In people with RRMS, we now know that variability can extend over many months, if not years. This means that EDSS progression is an unreliable indicator of permanent disability in RRMS, especially over shorter time scales.

- Are there sufficient participants in the study to detect what we are looking for? This is known as the power of the study to find the answer if it is there.

- Does the study go on for long enough to convince you that the effect is sustained and worthwhile in a chronic disease that may last for decades?

- Are potential sources of bias dealt with adequately? For example, does the trial describe how randomization occurred? Are there a lot of people lost to the final analysis? (It may be that everyone who did badly dropped out of the study, so it might look as though our treatment is better than it really is.) Most studies should be analysed according to 'intention to treat' methodology (ITT). This means that everyone randomized to that treatment group will be analysed at the end of the study as belonging to that group, even if they changed or stopped treatment. This methodology reduces bias and all trials should be scrutinized to make sure that the investigators do not 'lose' patients and make their results look better than they should be.

- Is the statistical analysis appropriate, and did the investigators specify what they were going to use as their main outcomes before the study started? If we use the 5% level as the standard level of statistical significance (so that we would expect one result in 20 to be down to pure chance), and the investigators performed 40 different analyses, we would expect two of these results to be positive, due to chance rather than treatment effect. If such analyses occurred, did the investigators adjust for this?

- What are the side effects of the treatment, and did people stop treatment because of side effects? Even if treatments work, they may be too toxic to justify routine use.

For more detailed evaluation of clinical trials methodology, the reader is referred to the CONSORT statement at *www.consort-statement.org*

In terms of MS-specific trials, there are examples of problems with virtually every trial ever conducted in the field, and the reader needs to evaluate the deficiencies to decide whether the broad conclusions are justified. One way of getting around the problems of individual trials is to combine the results of all published studies in the area, and see if the overall results are significant. This is known as meta-analysis, and can be an extremely valuable way of helping to interpret the data. The Cochrane collaboration was set up to do just this, and Cochrane reports tend to be useful overviews of the major research in any particular treatment. There are a number of Cochrane reviews which have been undertaken in the field of MS (refer to *www.thecochranelibrary.com*).

Part 2

Diagnosis

General points on making a diagnosis

Making a diagnosis of any neurological condition rests predominantly on obtaining a good history consistent with the clinical syndrome (ideally directly from the patient), looking for corroboration of findings on neurological examination that are consistent with the condition, and then using any investigations to add weight to the diagnosis one way or the other. A diagnosis cannot be made simply from an MR scan, or any other single part of the process. These days, the criteria by which a diagnosis of MS can be made have been generally agreed and published (Chapter 4), but medicine is often less clear-cut than published criteria, and uncertainty is part of everyday life.

It is important to consider the implications of finding diagnoses that may be unexpected, particularly when requesting investigations, which is why there are recommendations for patient counselling prior to many diagnostic tests. A good example of this is the requesting of cranial MRI in a young person with a mild self-limiting attack of vertigo or numbness. The commonest cause of vertigo is benign positional vertigo, yet one can never completely exclude a possible brainstem episode of inflammation, consistent with early MS. Is it better for a young person to know that they have lesions on cranial MRI that could lead to MS, even when most people may not consider treatment at that stage? The issue of how far to investigate minor symptoms varies with routine practice across the world and with any individual clinician's interpretation of the evidence that early treatment of clinically isolated syndromes (CIS) may lead to better long-term prognosis. Many people would judge that unless and until there is good long-term evidence that treating mild early episodes will have a beneficial effect on long-term welfare, then it may be better not to consider investigation unless something more severe were to occur. Some patients, once a diagnosis of MS has been made, remark that they would have preferred not to have been told about a possible diagnosis of MS at the earliest presentation of CIS, as the potential diagnosis of MS 'would have hung over me for years and ruined my life'. Other people are very much aware of possible diagnoses, can handle the possibilities psychologically, and feel angry if doctors are not fully open about the all of the diagnostic possibilities at every stage.

In the UK, the National Institute of Clinical Excellence (NICE) guidelines on the management of MS state the following:

'An individual should be informed of the potential diagnosis of MS, as soon as a diagnosis of MS is considered reasonably likely (unless there are over-whelming patient centred reasons for not doing so). This should occur before undertaking further investigations to confirm or refute the diagnosis …

When presenting with optic neuritis:

… If the diagnosis is confirmed as optic neuritis, without any other specific cause and possibly due to MS, the ophthalmologist should discuss the potential diagnosis with the individual (unless there are overwhelming patient-centred reasons for not doing so). A further referral to a neurologist for additional assessment should be offered.'

This is a controversial stance, particularly if there are delays in obtaining neurological opinions. Ideally, services should be configured to minimize potential anxiety, maximize patient welfare, and reduce the tendency to over-investigate symptoms that may be best managed in other ways.

Chapter 12

Sites of MS attack and clinically isolated syndromes

MS tends to present with specific syndromes, with a predilection to attack particular parts of the central nervous system, namely the optic nerves, the spinal cord and the brainstem. This is partly because these co-called eloquent areas contain a high density of important nerve pathways so that relatively small areas of inflammation may have significant clinical effects, which are readily noticed. However, they may also be other reasons to do with blood supply and expression of particular molecules that may play a role in the pathogenesis of MS.

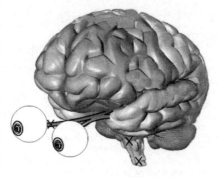

Fig. 12.1 MS tends to present in particular areas, especially the optic nerves, the brainstem, and the spinal cord (marked with x).

Typical presentations of clinically isolated syndromes

Optic neuritis

The optic nerves are particularly prone to inflammatory attack in MS. Optic neuritis is one of the commonest clinically isolated syndromes, and has an incidence of about 5 per 100,000 per year. Asymptomatic attacks of optic neuritis are also common, as demonstrated by finding abnormal visual evoked responses in people with MS who have not noticed any previous visual symptoms. The optic nerve meningeal sheath, which possesses most of the pain sensitive nerve fibres, is joined to the insertion of the eye muscles at the apex of the orbit. Eye movement can exacerbate the pain of optic neuritis, as muscle contraction pulls on the optic nerve sheath, already irritated by underlying inflammation. The characteristic features of optic neuritis are as follows:

Table 12.1 Symptoms of optic neuritis

- Unilateral
- Painful
- Visual blurring, colour desaturation, or complete blindness
- Relatively sudden onset—often either on waking or over a few hours or days
- Pain on eye movement
- Absence of any redness in the eye.

Table 12.2 Signs of optic neuritis

- Reduced visual acuity on Snellen chart
- Altered colour vision on Ishara colour plates
- Visual scotoma in 70% cases, often altitudinal
- Possible relative afferent papillary defect*
- Optic nerve head swelling in about 30% cases.

* Otherwise known as the Marcus Gunn phenomenon, tested by the swinging flashlight test. As the torch is shone into the unaffected eye, there is an ipsilateral and contralateral (consensual) constriction of the pupil. However, as the torch is then moved to the affected eye, instead of causing an ipsilateral constriction of the affected pupil, there appears to be a dilatation of that pupil, due to the relaxation of consensual constrictive response because the light signal entering the affected optic nerve (afferent signal) is reduced.

Although it is not uncommon for optic neuritis to sequentially affect one eye and then the other, sometimes with relatively little time between attacks, onset of simultaneous bilateral optic neuritis is very rare in Europe and North America (although relatively common in Japan), and should raise the possibility of other conditions including Leber's hereditary optic neuropathy (LHON), due to mutations in the mitochondrial genome.

Recovery of visual acuity is often the rule after the first attack of optic neuritis, with an average recovery time of around 2 months, although continued recovery can occur for at least 6 months. The extent of recovery is linked to the severity of the initial episode, so people with blindness are more likely to be left with residual visual field defects, alterations in colour perception, or residual reduced acuity.

Uhthoff (1889) originally described exercise-induced alteration of visual acuity in people with MS, due to reduced signal conduction with increased temperature along nerve fibres affected by myelin loss. Similar symptoms may be noticed by people with MS after a hot bath or in hot climates, especially during recovery from an episode of inflammation.

Repeated or severe attacks of optic neuritis may cause pallor of the optic disc on fundoscopy. This can be very difficult to spot, and is not a reliable sign unless extremely obvious, in which case visual acuity and colour vision are invariably affected.

Risk of developing MS after single episode of optic neuritis

Estimating risk can be difficult; in order to predict risk accurately we need access to large population studies over long periods with accurate case ascertainment and complete follow-up. Many studies examining the natural history of optic neuritis are retrospective, and there are very few studies with sufficient patients in the modern MRI era. With these caveats in mind, a typically quoted figure is around 50% of hospital based patients with optic neuritis will go on to develop MS after 15 years, although this figure may be lower in population surveys.

Early investigation can help in conveying risk of developing MS more accurately. The presence of oligoclonal bands in the cerebrospinal fluid is associated with increase risk of developing MS, as is the presence of abnormalities on cranial MRI. A normal cranial MRI at initial presentation of any clinically isolated syndrome has been associated with an approximate 20% risk of developing MS after 15 years, compared with 90% risk if the MRI is abnormal at presentation. Data from natural history studies in France suggest that it takes longer to develop MS if people present with optic neuritis rather than spinal cord or brainstem syndromes, although overall the CIS characteristics had little effect on subsequent progression. The most recent (10 year) results of the optic neuritis treatment trial suggest that most patients who develop MS after presenting with optic neuritis will have a relatively benign clinical course for at least 10 years, irrespective of initial MRI.

Treatment of optic neuritis

The largest acute treatment trial for any MS episode was the optic neuritis treatment trial, which randomized 389 patients with acute optic neuritis (and without known MS) to 1g methyl prednisolone intravenously for 3 days followed by 11 days of oral prednisolone (1mg/kg); oral prednisolone (1mg/kg) alone for 14 days; or oral placebo for 14 days. Initial follow-up was for 6 months, although 2-year follow-up was subsequently achieved in more than 90% of patients and the most recent publication has followed patients who developed MS over 10 years since initial presentation

Visual function recovered faster in the group receiving intravenous methyl prednisolone than in the placebo group. Although the differences between groups decreased with time, at 6 months, the group that received intravenous methyl prednisolone still had slightly better visual fields, contrast sensitivity (the 2 primary outcome measures) and colour vision, but not better visual acuity (which is less sensitive to change). The outcome in the oral prednisolone group did not differ from placebo. The authors also felt that treatment had most effect if given within the first 15 days after onset, and if visual acuity is worse than 6/12 on Snellen charts.

There was considerable controversy surrounding part of the analysis, which appeared to suggest that treatment with intravenous methyl prednisolone reduced the 2-year rate of developing MS, and in fact the risk of developing MS was increased in the oral prednisolone group. However, at 5 years, treatment had no significant effect on the development of MS, and earlier assumptions about risk of developing MS were misinterpretations of chance statistical significance (see Chapter 10).

Table 12.3 Treating optic neuritis

- High dose methyl prednisolone is treatment of choice.
- Low dose oral prednisolone (1mg/kg) no better than placebo.
- Consider treating if pain is major problem or if visual acuity <6/12.
- Little long-term effect of treatment at 6 months.
- Treatment most effective if given within 15 days from onset.

Transverse myelitis and spinal cord problems

The spinal cord, although smaller in volume than the brain itself, has such a high density of important signal pathways that probably the majority of new areas of inflammation will present clinically, whereas we know from studies using longitudinal MRI follow-up that many new lesions in parts of the brain can remain clinically silent. The precise combination of symptoms and signs associated with spinal cord problems will obviously depend of the site of inflammation within the cord.

One of the commonest symptoms in MS is sensory alteration, and may be the presenting feature of MS in up to 30–50% of cases. This may present with specific areas of numbness, sometimes being confused with the distribution of single peripheral nerves, or, more commonly, it may present with gradual evolution of sensory loss starting at one point and spreading either up or down over a period of days. For example, this may start in one foot, and spread up the leg onto the trunk and arm over a few days, getting up to the neck before spreading across to the other side. This type of presentation would be typical of a cervical cord lesion. Patients often describe burning or aching sensations, sometimes with trickling water feelings. This painful dysaesthesia is unfortunately quite common. Descriptions of 'tightness' or 'tight bands' are very characteristic of spinal cord problems. Most sensory levels in myelitis tend to be rather vague, persistent sharp cut-off should increase suspicion of alternative diagnoses.

Joint position sense travels from distal receptors via the posterior or dorsal spinal cord, so lesions in the dorsal cord can present with poor coordination in arm or leg. Typically when asked to hold their hands out in front of them with their eyes closed, the patient's fingers may move around in a type of wandering 'pseudoathetosis' because of the lack of feedback from joint position sense.

An important feature of spinal cord lesions is disturbance of bladder function, which must be asked about. Symptoms of urgency and frequency, with urge incontinence, are very common.

Initial involvement of the motor system is not uncommon, and carries a slightly poorer prognosis. Again, the site of the lesion determines the pattern, and patients may describe heavy legs, difficulty walking distances, or tripping over with foot dragging. Features suggestive of spinal cord motor involvement include a unilateral or bilateral increase in tone (usually in the legs), sometimes with sustained clonus at the ankle. Whereas up to 7–8 beats of clonus at the ankle can be within normal limits, any clonus at the patella should be a strong indication of an upper motor neurone problem. In keeping with an upper motor neurone or pyramidal type of problem, the pattern of weakness is important, with relative weakness of the leg flexors and the arm extensors. An easy way to remember this is to recall someone with a unilateral stroke, who may be able to walk with one leg extended (weakness of the flexors in the leg) and the arm on the same side flexed across the chest (weakness of the extensors of the arm). Mild upper motor neurone weakness may only be manifest as slight weakness of hip flexion with brisk reflexes on that side.

Testing tendon reflexes is an important part of the neurological examination, especially in the context of an ascending symmetrical numbness and weakness. A crucial differential diagnosis is acute Guillain–Barré syndrome or peripheral neuritis, which is due to inflammation in peripheral rather than central nerve pathways, therefore causing reduced or absent reflexes rather than the usual brisk reflexes typical of upper motor neurone syndromes. Plantar reflexes are often extensor in spinal cord syndromes, although not invariably so. Sometimes it is difficult to identify where the problem may be from the history, and one must weigh up the findings from both history and examination in order to locate the likely site of the lesion. It is important to always have in mind the question of 'where is the lesion?' in order to piece together difficult neurological presentations.

The term myelitis refers to any inflammation in the spinal cord. Transverse myelitis implies more extensive inflammation, affecting the majority of cross sectional area of the cord, although these terms are often used interchangeably. Occasionally hemi-cord syndromes may occur, including classical Brown–Sequard syndrome, causing ipsilateral pyramidal weakness and loss of joint position sense, but contralateral alteration of spinothalamic sensation (as the pain and temperature fibres have already crossed over shortly after entering the spinal cord).

Brainstem syndromes

In much the same way as spinal cord syndromes often present clinically because they occur in eloquent areas, so too brainstem syndromes reflect the particular part of the brainstem affected. Commoner symptoms of brainstem disturbance include: balance and coordination problems; vertigo (an abnormal sensation of movement, often room spinning in association with nausea, although the commonest cause of vertigo by far is a benign peripheral disturbance nothing to do with MS); and eye movement problems including double vision (diplopia).

One of the commonest brainstem features, especially in more advanced cases of MS, is an internuclear ophthalmoplegia (INO), due to demyelination in the medial longitudinal fasiculus, which connects the pontine gaze centre close to the VI nerve nucleus, with the contralateral III nerve nucleus (see Fig. 12.2). In order to move the eyes laterally on voluntary gaze, the pontine gaze centre drives the eyes towards the same side by stimulating the ipsilateral VI nerve (pulling on the lateral rectus muscle), and the contralateral medial rectus via the opposite III nerve. Demyelination in the signal transfer to the contralateral medial rectus will slow or abolish adduction of the contralateral eye, often with abducting nystagmus in the ipsilateral eye. This is best tested by rapid alternating eye movements whilst the head remains still. Occasionally patients may complain that 'one eye isn't keeping up with the other' or that they have to turn their head slowly in order to avoid double vision. More commonly, they may notice double vision, and sometimes they may not complain of any abnormality of vision, and these findings are only picked up on examination.

Many different combinations of cranial nerve abnormalities can be detected in brainstem inflammation, ranging from isolated cranial nerve palsies (such as lateral rectus palsy due to VI nerve problem), trigeminal neuralgia (a common problem, which, in a young person, should raise the suspicion of demyelination), facial palsy, and dysphagia. Deafness is probably under-recognized in MS, and vertigo is common. Isolated palsies of oculomotor (III), trochlear (IV), glossopharyngeal (IX), vagal (X), accessory (XI), and hypoglossal (XII) nerves are all incredibly rare and should raise the possibility of alternative diagnoses.

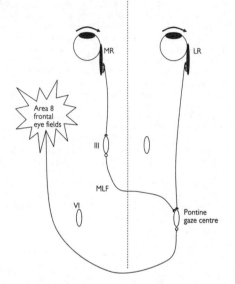

Fig. 12.2 Diagram of eye movement pathways in horizontal gaze. In this case the person is moving their eyes to their right. The signal starts in the frontal eye field, and is conveyed to the pontine gaze centre ipsilateral to the direction of the eye movement and then to the relevant motor nuclei and on to the muscles (medial rectus, MR, and lateral rectus, LR). In an internuclear ophthalmoplegia, demyelination in the medial longitudinal fasiculus (MLF) delays signal transmission and slows adduction of the contralateral eye.

There are a small number of rare clinical syndromes most often associated with demyelination, which raise the index of suspicion of MS if seen. These include facial myokymia, where the facial muscles are constantly moving with very fine flickers 'like a bag of worms'. This is not to be confused with the extremely common and usually benign fluttering of one eyelid, which if severe can be labelled as blepharospasm. Another rare phenomenon is ocular flutter, where either at rest or on movement, the eyes suddenly oscillate briefly for a fraction of a second.

Problems with coordination, ataxia, balance and slurred (so-called cerebellar) speech can be due to lesions within the cerebellum, within the brainstem, and are sometimes (with balance problems and ataxia) due to disturbance of connections to and from the cerebellum. Typically patients may have a wide-based gait, ataxia on finger-nose testing, or rapid alternating hand movements (dysdiadochokinesis), sometimes with tremor and slurred or scanning speech. Various types of nystagmus can also be detected and should be documented as occurring in the primary position (rare), or only on gaze in a particular direction (gaze-evoked), either horizontally or vertically. Although the classical teaching was that downbeat nystagmus is more typical of a lesion at the foramen magnum, and upbeat nystagmus is more typically found in lesions of the pons and midbrain, the advent of MRI has taught us that such classical teaching may not always be correct.

Differential diagnosis in MS and clinically isolated syndromes

Because inflammation and demyelination can affect virtually any part of the central nervous system, including the cortex, the list of differential diagnoses can be very long. However, in the majority of cases, especially after a second episode, the diagnosis of MS often becomes clear. Progressive syndromes can present more difficulty in diagnosis.

Some important questions in the diagnostic pathway are as follows:

- After full history and examination, can the syndrome be explained by a lesion in the central nervous system, or in the peripheral nervous system (in which case MS becomes much less likely)?
- Is the clinical syndrome typical of one seen in MS (e.g. optic neuritis or myelitis)?
- If the syndrome is slowly progressive, and the clinical picture could be explained by a single lesion, has the affected area been imaged?
- Are there any unusual features to the clinical picture or any of the investigations?
- How far do we need to go in order to exclude alternative diagnoses?
- Is the syndrome organic or non-organic (functional/hysterical), or possibly mixed?

Many of the progressive conditions listed in Table 12.4 can seemingly improve, sometimes giving the illusion of a relapsing condition with dissemination in time. These include certain meningiomas that may be hormonally responsive and alter with pregnancy; cavernous haemangiomas that may bleed and then resolve; cervical myelopathy when oedema surrounding a more acute deterioration may resolve; and cerebral lymphoma (which may classically apparently resolve radiologically after treatment with corticosteroids).

Another trap for the unwary is of two common conditions occurring either simultaneously or sequentially, leading to the illusion of dissemination in either time or space. For example, carpal tunnel syndrome and diabetic neuropathy, or Bell's palsy and cervical myelopathy. Usually these types of problem can be sorted out by careful history and examination, with ancillary tests if any doubt remains. Often some aspects of previous history will lead the clinician down specific diagnostic pathways, so previous episodes of blurred vision may suggest optic neuritis, but it is often unwise to place too much emphasis on vague history from many years previous.

A full social history is important in any consultation, provided the subject is approached with tact and sympathy. Social and environmental factors not only determine how any individual reacts to their physical condition, but they may also provoke abnormal illness behaviour masquerading as MS or other physical illness. Sometimes a question such as 'Have you been under much stress recently?' is helpful. It is not uncommon in neurology to find patients may exaggerate their weakness or disability in order to 'help the doctor'. Everyone responds to symptoms in different ways, and environmental pressures will influence how people cope with those symptoms.

Some other factors to consider are as follows:
- Employment history ('Do you enjoy your job?')
- Domestic surroundings ('Are you happily married? Do you have a partner?'), family pressures
- Exposure to people with MS (health professionals in particular may develop functional disorders mimicking diseases to which they have been exposed)
- Financial stresses
- Childhood unhappiness ('Did you grow up around here? Was it a happy childhood?')
- Recent bereavements (often best approached when enquiring about family history).

Table 12.4 Differential diagnoses of syndromes that could be confused with MS

Clinical syndrome	Main conditions to consider	Other features/hints
Progressive spinal cord syndromes	• Degenerative disease e.g. cervical myelopathy • Spinal tumours, e.g. meningioma, ependymoma • Spinal arteriovenous malformation • Developmental abnormalities including Arnold–Chiari malformation • Infections, including HTLV-1, HIV, TB, syphilis, Lyme disease • Hereditary spastic paraplegias • Spino–cerebellar ataxias (SCAs) • Cavernous haemangiomas • Subacute combined degeneration (vitamin B12 deficiency) • Paraneoplastic conditions	• LMN in hands, UMN features in legs • Consider meningiomas in middle-aged women • Can progress in stuttering fashion • Look for downbeat nystagmus • Risk factors, systemic signs of infection • Family history, normal MRI • Family history, genetic evaluation, LMN signs? • Can 'relapse' when they bleed, then improve • Can cause Lhermitte's phenomenon • Unusual in spinal cord, more common with cerebellar signs
Multifocal CNS presentation	• Vascular diseases including multiple emboli, endocarditis, myxoma • Systemic lupus erythematosus (SLE) • Anti-cardiolipin syndrome • Sjorgren's syndrome • Sarcoidosis • Cerebral lymphoma • Systemic or isolated CNS vasculitis • Behçet's disease • Progressive multifocal leukoencephalopathy • Disseminated secondary malignancy e.g. breast • Disseminated gliomatosis • Mitochondrial diseases • Adult-onset leukodystrophies (adrenoleukodystrophy, metachromatic leukodystrophy, Krabbe's disease, Pelizaeus-Merzbacher disease)	• Cranial MRI may help, consider echocardiogram • Look for systemic markers of inflammation • Can occur without SLE, history may be stroke-like • Sicca syndrome, diagnosis on salivary biopsy • Most commonly meningo-encephalitic syndrome • Can have dramatic response to corticosteroids • If systemic markers negative, may need biopsy • Ask about oral and genital ulceration • Due to JC virus in immunocompromised • Can get ring enhancing lesions in MS, biopsy? • Rare, will need biopsy diagnosis • Often basal ganglia involvement • Check long chain fatty acids, white cell enzymes, metachromatic granules, genetics

Table 12.5 Leukodystrophies, which can cause confusion in diagnosis of MS. All may have confluent areas on cranial MRI

Inherited disorder	Main features	Diagnostic tests
Adrenomyeloneuronopathy	• Most common form of X-linked adrenoleukodystrophy (X-ALD) • Young adults with progressive spastic paraparesis • 30% Addison's disease without neurological involvement • 70% will have adrenal insufficiency	• Gene identified, but mutations vary therefore no diagnostic genetic test • Increased very long chain fatty acids in plasma or fibroblasts • Bone marrow transplantation may help in early stages of disease • Lorenzo's oil may be helpful.
Pelizaeus–Merzbacher disease	• Usually presents in childhood with slowly progressive psychomotor retardation with ataxia, pyramidal involvement, and dystonia.	• Most commonly due to duplication of gene for proteolipid protein (PLP), which is only present in CNS, so peripheral nervous system is intact.
Metachromatic leukodystrophy	• Can occur in adult forms with cognitive and behavioural changes preceding motor changes, so may present to psychiatrists • Peripheral nerve involvement on nerve conduction studies	• Gene defects in aryl-sulphatase A (ASA), in sulphatide metabolism, • Diagnosis by measuring ASA in white cells with abnormal sulphatide (metachromatic material) storage on nerve biopsy.
Krabbe's disease (globoid cell leukodystrophy)	• Usually presents in childhood • Rapid motor (pyramidal and extrapyramidal) and cognitive deterioration with optic atrophy.	• Gene defect in Galactocerebroside beta galactosidase gene (GalC) • Diagnosis by GalC activity in white cells • May respond to bone marrow transplantation.

Specific demyelinating syndromes

Devic's disease

This condition is otherwise known as neuromyelitis optica (NMO), and is the combination of optic neuritis and, usually, extensive longitudinal myelitis. There is controversy over whether this represents a separate condition from conventional MS. It seems to be more common in the Far East, and does not appear to be the simple presence of optic neuritis with subsequent mild myelitis (very common), but is rather the presence of massive confluent areas of inflammation in the optic nerves (often both) and spinal cord, either simultaneously, or in rapid succession. Investigation often shows long swollen areas of inflammation in the spinal cord (with relatively normal brain MRI), and often the presence of neutrophils in the CSF, which is very uncommon in conventional MS. Oligoclonal immunoglobulin bands may be absent from the CSF. More recently the presence of specific antibodies has been described in Devic's disease, against a protein known as aquaporin–4, a water channel present on astrocytic end-feet. Prognosis is not good in Devic's disease, and high dose steroids may be complemented with plasmapheresis, or more recently rituximab in refractory relapsing cases.

Marburg's disease

This eponym is commonly attached to an unusually aggressive form of MS, which may be monophasic. It represents a syndrome rather than a specific condition, although there have been suggestions that some of these patients may have a mild background disorder of myelin, rendering them more susceptible to aggressive inflammatory attack. There is rapid accumulation of disability within very short periods—generally within 2 years, and often over a few months. Prognosis is poor and the difficulty lies in trying to recognize those individuals who could be classified in this group. It may represent up to 5% of early MS, depending on how it is classified. Various treatments have been tried, including plasma exchange, mitoxantrone, and alemtuzumab. Clinical trials of such aggressive disease are difficult to conduct, but in the future we should be aiming to attempt to identify such individuals with more confidence at an early stage, and then treat with aggressive therapy before too much disability has accumulated.

Acute disseminated encephalomyelitis (ADEM)

This is regarded as principally being a disease of childhood, with an acute demyelinating illness occurring shortly after an infection (usually viral) or immunization. Some of the most commonly implicated infections include measles (previously occurring at a rate of around 1 in 1,000 before routine immunization), mumps, rubella, varicella, influenza, and mycoplasma, although often no infectious agent may be identified. Immunizations against rabies, smallpox, measles and diptheria–tetanus–polio can also be associated with ADEM. Features of the condition include systemic disturbance (such as fever), often with large areas of confluent inflammation on MRI, CSF pleocytosis, and absent or only transiently positive oligoclonal bands in CSF. A relapsing or multiphasic disseminated encephalomyelitis

(MDEM) has also been described, but there is considerable controversy over whether this really represents a separate condition from MS. Indeed, it is often said that the differentiation between a clinically isolated syndrome and ADEM may be very difficult to make. Such controversy will continue to persist until specific diagnostic tests can be produced for each syndrome.

There is some evidence to suggest that ADEM may respond to plasma exchange if there is no improvement with high dose corticosteroids. If this is not available, or contraindicated for some reason, then the use of intravenous immunoglobulin has been described by some authors, although there is little good evidence for either.

Acute haemorrhagic leucoencephalitis

This is a thankfully very rare, more severe disease than ADEM, and is often fatal. It may simply be an extreme form of ADEM, in which microvascular haemorrhages occur, often with neurotrophils and lymphocytes in the CSF.

Chapter 13

Investigation for possible MS

Introduction and initial tests

The most important aspect of achieving a diagnosis for any neurological condition is to take a good history. When a person presents with definite episodes of neurological dysfunction, attributable to well-recognized MS syndromes, with evidence from a clear history and supported by clinical examination, there is a good argument for making a clinical diagnosis and not doing any tests at all. However, these days most people expect a scan, and it will help to determine prognosis, treatment options, and assist the patient in understanding their condition. The issue then remains as to how far one should go in trying to exclude other potentially rare causes for similar conditions. Most people would perform the tests in Table 13.1 when someone presents with an MS-type syndrome.

Table 13.1 Investigations for possible MS

- Full blood count, plasma viscosity.
- Blood glucose, electrolytes, liver function.
- Autoantibodies, including anti-nuclear factor, other relevant antibodies.
- Thyroid function.
- Vitamin B12.
- MRI head (together with spinal cord if presenting with spinal syndrome).

Magnetic resonance imaging (MRI) in MS

This type of scan is an extremely sensitive method for picking up areas of abnormality within the brain, and has revolutionized the diagnosis of MS. However, the reader should remember that cranial MRI is not specific for MS, even when various criteria are applied to improve specificity. Above all, the diagnosis of MS should **never** be made on the basis of cranial MRI alone. When taken in conjunction with an appropriate clinical history and neurological examination, then MRI can be extremely helpful.

MRI is essentially a method of imaging magnetized protons, and is therefore very sensitive to detecting abnormal water composition in parts of the brain. Signal can be obtained in a number of ways, and the characteristic changes seen in MS are best demonstrated using either T2-weighted or proton–density sequences. Lesions seen on such scans do not represent specific pathology, but rather a mixture of different pathological processes, including oedema, astrocytic scarring, demyelination, and inflammation. The site and shape of lesions can help to improve the specificity of MR scanning; in other words, the chances that the changes seen are related to MS rather than an alternative pathology. A pragmatic agreement on the type of changes providing both specificity and sensitivity can be found in the agreed diagnostic criteria in Chapter 4. If there are a large number of lesions, with a mainly paraventricular distribution, with some lesions in the posterior fossa, and others in a subcortical distribution, then the chances are relatively high that this will be MS. In technical terms, the sensitivity and specificity are around 70–75%.

MRI is a technology that is developing rapidly, and machines are becoming more powerful. Most of the data mentioned above relates to machines ranging from 0.5–1.5 Tesla (a measurement of magnetic strength achieved in machine design). With new generation 3 Tesla machines becoming available, the chances of detecting abnormal signal which does not reflect MS pathology increases greatly. Even using the relatively specific MRI criteria mentioned earlier, if we were to rely on MRI to make a diagnosis, we would be wrong in 25% of people. This becomes much more of a problem when investigating people over the age of 50, when high signal lesions become more common. This is also true when other conditions such a hypertension and diabetes are present. It is thought that most of these lesions represent small areas of vascular damage, which can be indistinguishable from small MS lesions. It is under these circumstances that additional investigations such as cerebrospinal fluid (CSF) analysis may be necessary.

Another commonly used MRI technique is the intravenous injection of gadolinium DTPA (gd-DTPA) contrast agent, which will demonstrate areas of breakdown in the normally integral blood–brain-barrier (BBB). Studies have shown that gd-DTPA contrast enhancement is usually the first event in the development of acute lesions and often persists for up to 6–8 weeks after an initial episode of BBB breakdown. Such studies have demonstrated episodes of contrast enhancement on MRI that wax and wane, often without concurrent clinical events. Again, higher doses of gd-DTPA will demonstrate more activity, but the role of so-called triple dose gadolinium in the routine management of MS patients is unclear. Many centres do not routinely perform gd-DTPA contrast injection unless patients are part of a research project, or there is some other reason for knowing whether a lesion is new or old.

Although MRI has been used to monitor disease activity (usually by counting lesion load, new enhancing lesions or, more recently, calculating atrophy based on accurate outlining of brain substance using specific orientation techniques) the correlation between clinical disability and most MRI measures is poor. This may partly be due to the poor clinical measures in use over the last 20 years, and because a lot of disability is due to spinal cord disease rather than brain disease. There is certainly a better correlation between spinal cord diameter and measures such as the EDSS, which relies heavily on mobility, especially in the middle portion of the scale. The presence of so-called 'black holes' on T1-weighted images also correlates better with disability and axonal loss than more conventional T2-weighted images.

Other research techniques include magnetic resonance spectroscopy (MRS), which has the capacity to generate chemical spectra (graphs of chemical composition) within designated areas of brain. This may improve the specificity with which areas of abnormality related to demyelination may be distinguished from other pathologies such as a tumour. Other techniques such as diffusion weighted imaging (DWI) and magnetization transfer ratio (MTR) are still being evaluated with respect to their value in routine imaging of MS patients. It is hoped that in the near future we may be able to use imaging to distinguish the separate processes of BBB breakdown, demyelination and remyelination/repair. Such capacity would lead to greatly facilitated tailoring of individual patient treatment regimes, as well as monitoring of disease processes. At the moment, however, most people with MS will have a single scan at diagnosis, and there is no proof that routine monitoring using MRI provides any additional advantages in terms of disease management. MRI provides one tool in the overall evaluation of patients, but ultimately it has not yet provided the surrogate measure that might facilitate better patient care; we are still treating people, and not brain scans.

Examples of MR images

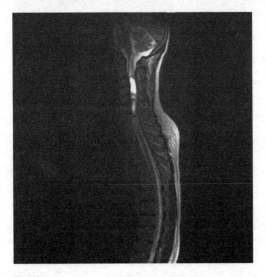

Fig. 13.1 Spinal cord syndrome not due to MS, in this case an ependymoma which has bled.

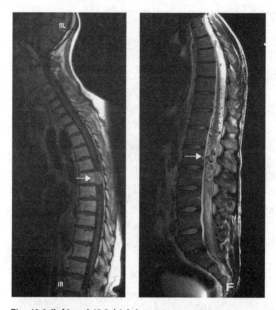

Figs 13.2 (left) and 13.3 (right) Spinal cord syndromes not due to MS. 13.2 due to thoracic meningioma (arrow) and 13.3 due to arteriovenous malformation (arrow).

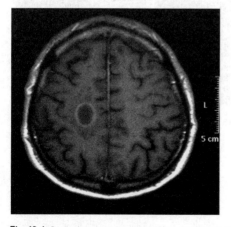

Fig. 13.4 Cerebral syndrome mimicking MS, in this case due to secondary tumour.

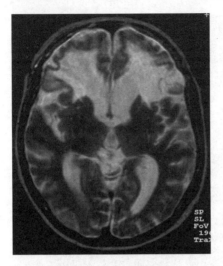

Fig. 13.5 Large confluent abnormalities in the frontal lobes not due to MS, in this case traumatic head injury.

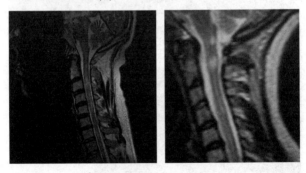

Fig. 13.6 Cervical spinal cord syndromes due to MS, with high signal in spinal cord.

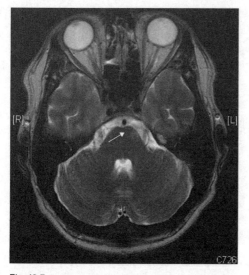

Fig. 13.7 Single area of high signal in the brainstem due to clinically isolated syndrome.

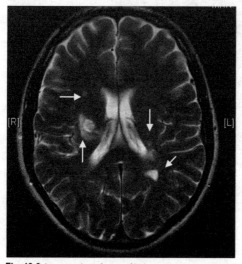

Fig. 13.8 Large number of areas of high signal consistent with MS.

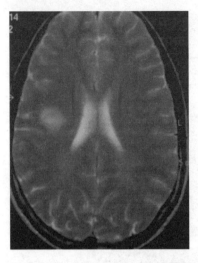

Fig. 13.9 Abnormal cranial MRI in early MS with large single lesion in right frontal area.

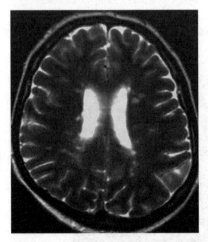

Fig. 13.10 Cranial MRI from someone with established MS, showing numerous high signal lesions.

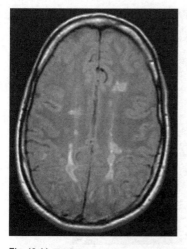

Fig. 13.11 FLAIR sequence showing cranial MRI from someone with MS, demonstrating confluent periventricular lesions.

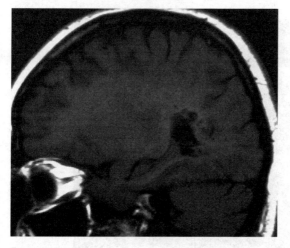

Fig. 13.12 T1 weighted sequence from someone with MS, showing 'holes' in the corpus callosum.

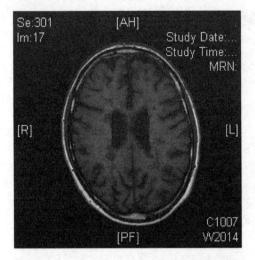

Fig. 13.13 T1 weighted MRI sequence showing 'holes' in a periventricular distribution.

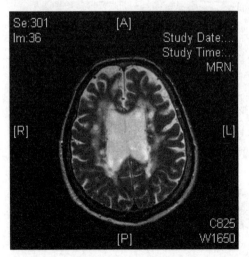

Fig. 13.14 T2 weighted MRI showing global atrophy of brain in advanced MS. This is especially obvious in the ventricles, with numerous high signal lesions in a paraventricular distribution. Some of these areas are confluent.

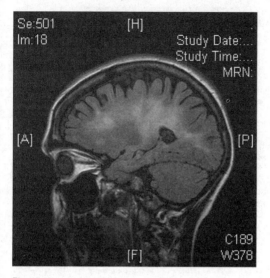

Fig. 13.15 FLAIR MRI sequence showing large confluent areas of abnormality in advanced progressive MS with global cerebral atrophy.

Lumbar puncture and cerebrospinal fluid (CSF) analysis

With the widespread introduction of MRI, the use of CSF analysis in the diagnosis of MS has diminished. However, it remains an essential tool in the investigation of many cases of potential MS, particularly if alternative diagnoses are being considered.

When a lumbar puncture is being considered, it is important to counsel the patient about potential risks and benefits. In experienced hands, lumbar puncture under local anaesthetic is a relatively painless procedure, with usually little in the way of complications. A post lumbar puncture headache may occur in up to 10% of cases, typically inducing headache and vomiting on standing or sitting, which may persist for some days. This complication is due to low CSF pressure, and meningeal oedema, which can be visualized with contrast enhanced MRI, although this is not clinically necessary in the vast majority of cases. Headache risk can be minimized using non-cutting lumbar puncture needles, with small diameter, as well as asking patients to drink large volumes of fluid after the procedure. Most people would recommend at least 4 hours' bed rest after the procedure, although recent evidence seems to suggest this is probably unnecessary. If a post lumbar puncture headache does occur, it is best treated with an epidural blood patch, where the patient's own blood is withdrawn, and injected into the epidural space by an experienced anaesthetist.

When a lumbar puncture is performed to obtain CSF, a sample of venous blood should also be drawn to send to the laboratory for blood glucose estimation, and to facilitate the paired evaluation of immunoglobulin (IgG) synthesis in blood and CSF. Intrathecal IgG synthesis is typical of MS, probably occurring in more than 95% of cases (see Fig. 13.16). Serum and CSF should be subject to electrophoresis on agarose gels with iso-electric focusing in order to look for the presence or absence of oligoclonal IgG bands. Oligoclonal bands present in the CSF but not in the serum suggest intrathecal synthesis, and an immune response specific to the CNS. This is the typical pattern seen in MS, although initially both serum and CSF may contain similar bands (so-called mirror pattern), which in time may change to an intrathecal synthesis pattern. As in the case of MRI, even if intrathecal immunoglobulin synthesis is demonstrated, this is not specific for MS and can be found in a number of other conditions. These include vasculitis, paraneoplastic syndromes, neurosarcoidosis, as well as infections and complications thereof, neurodegenerative disorders, neuropathies and myopathies, as well as psychiatric disorders and narcolepsy. However, the presence of oligoclonal bands does raise the index of suspicion for MS, and if combined with characteristic changes on MRI, then the chances of the condition being MS are around 97%.

In addition to expecting to see oligoclonal bands in people affected by MS for a number of years, there are a small minority of people with true oligoclonal band negative MS, who appear to have a relatively good prognosis. These people are rare, and the absence of oligoclonal bands after a number of years raises the strong possibility of alternative diagnoses.

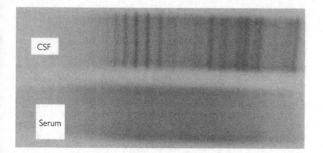

Fig. 13.16 CSF isoelectric focussing for oligoclonal band detection. Bands are seen in the CSF but not in the serum, suggesting local immune response in the CSF due to proliferation of specific clones of inflammatory B lymphocytes.

As well as analysis for oligoclonal bands, CSF should be analysed for total protein and cell count. Occasionally, total protein is slightly elevated in MS, but levels above 1g/L are rare. Similarly, slight lymphocytosis may be seen, especially in active disease, although levels above 100 cells/mm^3 are rare. Neutrophils are also unusual in CSF from MS patients except in Devic's disease (Chapter 12). Unexpected CSF findings should again raise the index of suspicion for alternative diagnoses, and may lead to the need for additional CSF analysis such as cytology or specific microbiological analysis.

Evoked potentials

When normally insulated nerve fibres lose their insulation, which occurs in MS due to loss of the myelin sheath, they conduct electrical impulses less well. This delay in signal conduction velocity can be measured in various pathways in humans, and can be used to provide evidence for dissemination of areas of demyelination in the central nervous system. These techniques can also be used to investigate symptoms in the absence of signs on clinical examination.

By measuring conduction of a signal from the eyes (visual evoked response), ears (auditory evoked response) and arms and legs (somatosensory evoked response) to the brain, we can establish any delay in the normal conduction time, and look at the size of the evoked potential, which might indicate loss of nerve fibres or temporary conduction block. It is also possible to stimulate motor pathways in the brain using transcranial magnetic stimulation, in order to test the motor pathways. Again, with the emergence of MRI, the use of evoked potentials has diminished, although visual evoked responses in particular are important in confirming dissemination of lesions by often providing proof of previous optic neuritis, even if someone has been asymptomatic from the visual perspective. Figure 13.17 shows a typical evoked response.

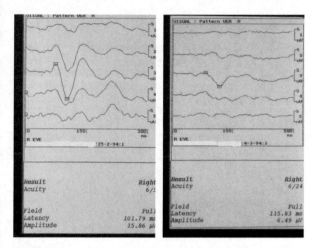

Fig. 13.17 Visual evoked response (VER) from the right eye of a patient during their episode of optic neuritis. The VER is measured over the occipital cortex in response to a visual stimulus of a black and white chequerboard pattern on a screen. This produces a detectable wave, known as the P100, as the latency (delay in signal conduction between eye and brain) is usually around 100ms. The record on the left was taken on the day that the patient started to get symptoms, when the visual acuity was normal (6/5) and the latency was also within the normal range (101.79ms). A few days later, the signal was rapidly reduced (with an amplitude less than half of the previous response), and a prolonged latency of 115.83ms. The clinical reflection of this was a reduced visual acuity of 6/24.

Conveying the diagnosis

The diagnostic phase has been described as a time of anxious waiting and a crucial period for people with MS. The delay between presenting symptoms, diagnostic tests, and receipt of results has been reported as a main area of complaint by people with MS. The lack of sensitivity in communicating the diagnosis has also been identified as an area of concern. The setting and circumstances of the disclosure of the diagnosis may have a direct effect on how a person reacts to the diagnosis.

Consultant neurologists, GPs, and junior hospital medical staff are the three main types of physicians involved in communicating the diagnosis of MS. Consultant neurologists have been identified as having a lead role in disclosing the diagnosis due to their knowledge of the disease and its effects. It has been suggested that GPs may be ideally placed to relay the diagnosis as they often have close personal knowledge of the patient. However, the fact that most GPs have limited experience or knowledge of MS can be a disadvantage to this approach.

Breaking bad news

It is important to recognize that receipt of a diagnosis of MS is 'bad news' as the information is likely to alter how the person views their future. It is essential that communication of the diagnosis is balanced with an emphasis on hope and realistic positivism.

Points to remember when communicating bad news are summarized in Tables 14.1, 14.2, and 14.3.

Table 14.1 Communicating bad news: key points

- Difficult news can never sound good.
- The honesty of the message should never be changed to improve acceptability.
- It is important to explain the situation to reduce uncertainty about the future, to enable appropriate adjustments to be made.
- It is important to encourage and support hope that is realistic to the person's circumstances.
- For some people the news may be so upsetting that they block out hearing anything being said—in this case the interaction may be short and a further meeting should be arranged.

Table 14.2 Flow chart for breaking bad news

Do I have all the facts/information?

⇩

Has the patient had the opportunity to have another person present?

⇩

Is a quiet room available? If not, maximize privacy.

⇩

Have I asked 'What do you understand about your condition so far?'

⇩

Give information slowly and gently, avoiding medical terminology.

⇩

Ask if further information is wanted at this time.

⇩

Encourage patient to express their feelings and any concerns.

⇩

Summarize and plan follow-up. Future availability is essential.

⇩

Communicate with other team members and document in notes.

Adapted from *Breaking Bad News to Adults*, University College London Hospital, 2006.

Table 14.3 Principles of good communication in healthcare

In any communication the healthcare professional should:

Principle	Comment
Communicate in a suitable environment, usually a quiet area or room free from distraction or interruption.	Privacy and quiet are important.
Seek agreement from the person with MS that anyone present can be there and ensure as far as possible that anyone s/he wants present is there.	Consider especially students and family.
Start by asking what the person knows or believes already.	Establishes expectations.
Establish the nature and extent of the information that the person wishes to receive.	Establishes expectations.
Consider carefully the balance between the benefits and the risks associated with giving each item of information.	Once given information cannot be withdrawn.
Tailor the communication to the person's: • Specific situation • Communicative and cognitive abilities • Culture.	Makes information relevant.
Limit information given to that within their own knowledge, referring on to others as necessary for more detailed information.	Do not give information if uncertain about it.
Clarify specifically any options and choices the person may need to choose, specifying: • Likely outcomes of each choice • Benefits and risks of each choice.	Both in diagnosis and treatment.
Offer back-up with information being given: • In different ways (e.g. written leaflets, tapes) • By different people (e.g. specialist nurse) • At another time (e.g. follow-up appointment).	Information is often forgotten.
Inform the person with MS about any recommended local or national sources of further information, including employment and voluntary sector sources.	Allows person with MS to follow-up and take more control.
Consider need for emotional support during process, especially if the information might be stressful, and arrange emotional support if needed.	Should be considered an intrinsic part of the process.
Document in notes and inform other health staff closely involved what has been communicated, especially the GP.	Ensures consistency over time and across settings.

Reproduced with permission from *NICE guidelines for the management of MS in primary and secondary care*, Table 2, p.19, 2003

Providing support at the time of diagnosis

The receipt of a diagnosis of MS causes emotional trauma, and individuals may respond in a number of ways. The care received at the time of diagnosis is central to the adaptation processes as information given and received may impact on the person with MS for the rest of their life. Appropriate support, information, education and guidance can help people adapt to the impact of the diagnosis. People with MS want a clear, accurate diagnosis, access to appropriate support, information, and continuing education at and around the time of diagnosis (Table 14.4).

While this support is often fulfilled by specialist MS nurses, it is important that all team members should be competent in offering emotional support. The NICE guidelines suggest that each person and team in contact with the person with MS should consider actively the need for emotional support by the person with MS and should endeavour to meet that need directly or through referral to any available suitable resource.

At the time of diagnosis, emotional support should be backed up by written information. Charitable bodies such as the MS Society or MS Trust provide information packs for people who are newly diagnosed (refer to Chapter 32 for details on useful resources/websites). These should be offered to all people. In addition, helpline telephone numbers and the names and contact telephone numbers of members of the MS team at the hospital should be given.

Research has shown that the newly diagnosed person may have a multitude of needs, including living with an uncertain future, experiencing wide symptomatic variability, and needing emotional, spiritual and psychosocial support. Specialist MS nurses and allied health professionals are well placed to provide support at this crucial time. A model of care that summarizes what a patient and their family need during this difficult time is summarized in Table 14.5.

Provision of clear, accurate evidence-based information can help to enable the person and their families to feel informed and supported. This approach can be initiated at the time of diagnosis through information sessions. The health professional can listen to fears and worries, assess the patient's perception of the disease, correct misconceptions, explain the pathology of existing symptoms, and make appropriate referrals to meet individual needs. It is important to recognize that physical function, social interaction and emotional wellbeing can impact upon how the person with MS and their family cope and adapt to the diagnosis. By understanding this, the health professional can introduce the concept of self-management to the person with MS (refer to Chapter 18).

Table 14.4 Key issues for people at time of diagnosis

- Certain, clear diagnosis
- Appropriate support at diagnosis
- Access to information
- Continuing education.

Adapted from *Standards of healthcare for people with multiple sclerosis* 1997. London: Multiple Sclerosis Society of Great Britain and Northern Ireland and The National Hospital for Neurology and Neurosurgery.

Table 14.5 Support at time of diagnosis

- E = education (about the disease, its course, symptomatic management and psychosocial implications)
- A = adaptation (adjustment, modifying lifestyle, setting priorities, promoting self-care)
- S = support (counselling, providing information on support groups, help in obtaining entitlements)
- E = enhancement (self-care, improvement of coping skills, facilitation of communication re: needs/concerns).

Adapted from Halper J. The needs of people who are newly diagnosed with multiple sclerosis. *MS Management* 1999; 1–4

Part 3

Treatment options

Treatments that may affect the underlying course of MS

Introduction

In considering the options, the reader is referred to Chapter 10, which outlines some of the major issues in deciding about treatment effectiveness. This is an area of very active research, and the following points are worth remembering:

- Clinical trial methodology is moving on at a slower pace than the development of new drugs, but it is moving. This means that though some of the older treatments (such as azathioprine) have not been subject to the same degree of scrutiny as newer agents, it does not necessarily mean that newer treatments are superior.

- Much heat and relatively little light is created when pharmaceutical companies compete with similar products in the same market, sometimes generating clinical trials that provide more in the way of marketing opportunities than serious scientific research.

- Whilst there are around 150 products under evaluation in the drug development pipeline, the picture is emerging that we will probably have to put up with more in the way of potentially serious side effects if we want to see good efficacy.

- Most of the evidence to date suggests that if we want to use drugs acting on the immune system to treat MS, then we will need to intervene at a stage before significant disability has accumulated. The size of effect obtained by any immunomodulatory drugs in the later phases of progressive disease is probably not worth the risk of benefit likely to be derived from their use.

- There is an urgent need to develop treatments for progressive disease, which are not likely to be drugs working on the immune system. Most progression appears to be mainly neurodegenerative in nature, which may benefit from a different approach to drug treatment. In the future, we may need to use combinations of neuroprotective agents, immunomodulatory agents, and techniques to encourage natural repair processes.

Over the last few years the term 'immunomodulatory' has become increasingly used to define milder treatments, without obvious profound immunosuppression (e.g. beta interferons). More powerful drugs, such as cytotoxic agents that target all dividing cells including cells of the immune system, are often referred to as immunosuppressive.

Beta-interferon

The initial rationale behind the use of beta-interferon was based on the theory that MS has a viral aetiology and that interferons (IFN), being naturally occurring cytokines, are produced in vivo by cells in response to viral infection. This led to the first trials using interferon-gamma (IFN-γ) in a group of MS patients in the mid 1980s. The observation of an adverse increase in relapse rate secondary to IFN-γ led to the cautious introduction of IFN-β as a possible immunomodulatory agent, on the basis that it was known to be a natural inhibitor of IFN-γ. As a result of a few promising initial small studies, further randomized trials were undertaken to fully assess its effect in MS.

There are two main beta-interferons currently licensed for use, having been shown to have some beneficial effect by reducing the relapse rate in MS. IFN-β1a has an amino acid sequence identical to native human IFN-β and differs from IFN-β1b in being glycosylated. The two licensed forms of this agent are Rebif ®, given subcutaneously three times a week, and Avonex®, given by intramuscular injection once weekly. These two agents are both produced in Chinese hamster ovary cells with identical amino acid sequences to the natural IFN-β, but differ from each other in their stabilizer and buffer properties, as well as route of administration. In contrast, IFN-β1b is cloned in bacteria and has a single amino acid substitution that differentiates it from native human IFN-β. It is given as a subcutaneous injection every other day. The most common side effects of IFN-β are influenza-like symptoms and local injection site reactions. Other less common side effects include nausea and vomiting, rashes, raised liver enzymes, mood changes, and convulsions.

No clear mechanism of action has been proven, although in addition to its antiviral action, interferon beta also has been shown to dampen immune-augmented effects. IFN-γ augments expression of MHC proteins on macrophages, a major participant in inflammatory foci within the brain in MS, as well as inducing protein expression on astrocytes. IFN-β counteracts these actions, down regulating class II MHC antigen expression, lessening antigen presentation to T-cells and antagonising the release of tumour necrosis factor and other possible toxins by activated macrophages. In vitro, IFN-β has also been shown to restore deficient suppressor function of T-cells, often seen in MS patients. It is possible therefore that IFN-β is working through these channels to alter the immune response, and produce its therapeutic effect.

Table 15.1 Different forms of beta interferon

Available types of beta-interferon for treating MS:

IFN-β1b (Betaferon®)—for subcutaneous injection, 300mcg alternate days.

IFN-β1a (Avonex®)—for intramuscular injection 30mcg once weekly.

IFN-β1a (Rebif®)—for subcutaneous injection 22 or 44mcg three times/week.

Beta interferon in relapsing-remitting MS

The first major randomized phase III study of beta-interferon for the treatment of relapsing-remitting multiple sclerosis (MS) was published in 1993 by the *interferon beta-1b (IFNB)* MS Group. This study was a multicentre, randomized, double-blind, placebo-controlled trial of IFN-β administered by subcutaneous injection every other day. Entry criteria included an EDSS of 0–5.5 and at least two exacerbations in the previous 2 years. A total of 372 patients were recruited, one third receiving placebo, and one third each receiving IFN-β either 1.6 million international units (MIU) or 8 MIU. The trial reported a statistically significant reduction in relapse rate of about 30%. However, this study has been criticised for its lack of intention-to-treat analysis as well as its high dropout rate. Data from patients who withdrew was censored and it is difficult to explain how more patients were available for follow-up after 3 years than 2. In addition, 20% of patients self-reported exacerbations without neurological confirmation. If these are excluded from the analysis, the data is no longer statistically significant. The trial also failed to show any significant effect on the secondary outcome measure of disability over the course of the 2 year study period, despite an encouraging improvement on the number of new inflammatory lesions on cranial MRI. This trial was initially conducted for 2 years and then extended in an unblinded fashion to 5 years. However, statistical power at 5 years was affected due to high dropouts, especially in the placebo group, which had a disproportionately high exacerbation rate and MRI lesion load compared with the treatment group dropouts.

The second significant trial published in 1996 by Jacobs *et al.* with the MS Collaborative Research Group (MSCRG) administered weekly intramuscular IFNβ-1a injections, again in a double-blind, randomized, placebo-controlled multicentre trial, in 301 recruited patients with a baseline EDSS of 1.0–3.5 and at least two exacerbations in the previous 3 years. This study differed from the IFN-β group study by using disability as its primary outcome measure (determined as deterioration by ≥1.0 point on the EDSS for at least 6 months). Despite claiming that time to progression was significantly delayed in the treated group, only 172/301 completed the 2 year period as the trial was terminated prematurely. Analysis of those completing the full 2 years showed an insignificant effect on disability progression. In addition, all recruited patients had a very low disability scale score, and at this level the degree of inter-observer variability is high. As a secondary outcome, however, the trial did confirm a significant reduction in relapse rate with the high dose treatment group.

The Prevention of Relapses and Disability by IFN-β1a in MS Study Group (PRISMS) is one of the largest studies, being multicentre, multinational, and recruiting 560 patients with an EDSS score of 0–5.0. Patients were randomly assigned subcutaneous IFNβ-1a at one of two dosages or placebo, for 3 times a week for 2 years. The primary outcome measure was relapse count over the course of the study. Once again, a significant effect on relapse reduction was observed. This clinical effect was reported to continue for both doses at 4 year follow-up. Prolongation in time to progression of disability was also noted. However, the Cochrane collaboration calculated a weighted mean of –0.25 when combining data from both the IFN-β MS group and the PRISMS trial, and such a small degree of change is of questionable clinical importance.

Beta interferon in secondary progressive MS

Despite the above trials reporting a reduction in relapse rate, the effect of interferon on disease progression remains unclear. Therefore, in an attempt to assess its effect upon disability, several large studies have looked at the efficacy of IFN-β, both 1a and 1b, in SPMS patients. The most widely reported are the European Study Group (using IFN-β1b) and the SPECTRIMS study (Secondary Progressive Efficacy Clinical Trial of Rebif® (IFN-β1a) in MS).

The European group studied 718 patients for up to 3 years with a primary outcome measure of time to disease progression. This again was a multicentre, randomized, double-blind, placebo-controlled trial, and included patients with a baseline EDSS of 3.0–6.5 with SPMS for at least 6 months. The patients received either placebo or 8 MIU of IFN-β1b by subcutaneous injection every other day. Treatment was discontinued prematurely in 220 patients (approx 30% of each group). The study concluded that the treated group had a significantly longer time to disease progression (EDSS 1.0–point) than placebo. Interestingly, however, a large proportion of patients experienced superimposed relapses, with this subgroup showing a more pronounced treatment effect and a reduction in relapse rate; not surprising given the experience in the RRMS trials. The result of the North American Betaferon secondary progressive trial was reported in 2000 and, in contrast to the European study, showed no treatment effect up to 8 MIU of IFN-β1b administered every other day. Therefore it has been suggested that the results of the European group reflected the transient reduction in EDSS experienced after relapses rather than overall progression. The SPECTRIMS study also failed to show a significant delay in patients treated with IFN-β1a given by subcutaneous injection 3 times a week. A total of 571 (92.4%) patients were followed up for 3 years. This group of patients also had a baseline EDSS of 3–6.5 but analysis of the subgroups revealed that patients in the relapsing group were less likely to progress, with a reduction in relapse rate; but that for the non-relapsing group, the effect was not significant.

Thus to date there is no good evidence for the effect of beta-interferon on delaying the progression of MS in the absence of relapses. There is no doubt that it has a modest effect upon the reduction of relapse rate; however, this does not seem to translate into prevention of clinical progression and disability.

Beta interferon and MRI

Many trials have also assessed the impact of treatment upon MRI findings and consistently report decreases in burden of disease (assessed by total area of T2 and proton density lesions) with treatment groups compared with placebo. One of the first trials to report such an effect was by the IFNB MS Study Group, with the placebo group showing a 17.1% increase in mean lesion area over 3 years versus a 6.2% decrease in the high dose treatment group. Subgroup analysis of 52 patients undergoing serial scans every 6 weeks for 2 years showed a 75% reduction in the rate of new lesion formation in the high dose group. The PRISMS trial reported similar results, from 550 RRMS patients, having scans every 6 months. Over the two years the interferon groups showed a decrease in burden of disease, with clear dose effect, by 3.8% (for higher dose) compared with the placebo group which showed an increase of approximately 11%.

The Once Weekly Interferon for MS Study Group (OWIMS) assessed a primary outcome measure of the number of combined unique active lesions at 24 weeks detected by MRI scanning (i.e. PD/T2 or T1-Gd activity). They also used this study to assess the effect of lower and less frequent doses of subcutaneous injections of IFN-β1a. A total of 293 patients were recruited, one third each receiving either placebo or one of two doses of interferon. They reported a statistically significant reduction in all MRI measures with the higher dose group (44mcg), but with lesser effects on clinical measures, being reduced but not significant.

Similar studies have been performed in the secondary progressive group of patients. The European Study Group analysed MRI to determine the effect of treatment on the pathological evolution of the disease in secondary progressive patients with IFN-β1b. Again, a statistically significant difference was seen between the placebo and treated group, with an increase in total lesion volume of 15% in the former, but a decrease of 2% in the latter. Interestingly, however, serial MRI in a subgroup of 95 patients showed no significant effect of treatment on cerebral atrophy, with both groups having a significant and progressive decrease in cerebral volume.

A meta-analysis of the predictive value of gadolinium (Gd)-enhanced MRI for relapse rate and changes in disability has been performed, which concluded that the best relapse rate predictor was the mean number of Gd enhancing lesions in serial scans, but not in one scan alone. No scans were predictive of the change in EDSS.

Early intervention with beta interferon

The finding of reduction in relapse rate with no clear effect on disease progression has led to a reassessment of the relationship between inflammation and degeneration. This has led to a change in the approach to MS and contributed towards the theory that, perhaps by targeting the very initial event, thus preventing the initial damage, disease progression will be halted. Many studies have demonstrated that axonal damage occurs in both acute and active chronic MS lesions. Therefore, with this in mind, it would seem logical to target clinically isolated syndrome (CIS) patients and thus reduce time to second relapse and possible formation of further inflammatory plaques, delaying or even preventing the onset of clinically definite MS (CDMS). Three published studies have looked at the treatment of interferon in the very early stages of MS. The ETOMS study (Early Treatment of Multiple Sclerosis with Rebif®) randomized 309 patients to receive placebo or IFN-β1a (Rebif®) at 22mcg as a weekly subcutaneous injection over 2 years. The selected patients had had a first clinical episode suggestive of demyelinating disease within the previous 3 months and abnormal brain MRI findings suggestive of MS. The primary outcome was the proportion of patients converting to clinically definite MS. The study reported significantly prolonged time to conversion to CDMS in the treated group, stating a 31% reduction in the risk of conversion compared to placebo. This trial was undertaken prior to the OWIMS and PRISMS results and therefore only used a low dose of interferon. If, as suggested, there is a dose effect, this clearly needs to be repeated at higher doses.

Jacobs *et al.* performed a similar study in 383 patients who had a first acute clinical demyelinating event and an abnormal MRI (thus high risk of developing CDMS). They were randomized to receive either placebo, or weekly intramuscular injections of IFN-β1a (30mcg). The end points were the development of CDMS and changes in findings on the MRI of the brain. Again, this group showed that during the 3 years of follow-up, treatment with IFN-β1a reduced the probability of developing CDMS. As with other MRI data, the treatment group also had a significant relative reduction in the volume of brain lesions compared with placebo. This trial was terminated early after a preplanned interim efficacy analysis. However, as a result, the question of whether treatment with beta interferon will prevent the onset of secondary progressive disease remains unanswered.

The most recent study reported the use of IFN-β1b (Betaferon®) in people with a clinically isolated syndrome and two clinically silent MRI lesions. People were randomized to 250mcg IFN-β1b (292) or placebo (176) and followed until they developed another clinical syndrome (occurred in 45% of patients on placebo) or fulfilled the McDonald criteria for a diagnosis of MS (occurred in 85% of patients on placebo). The hazard ratio of developing MS with IFN use was 0.5 for clinical MS and 0.54 if McDonald criteria were applied.

The role of neutralizing antibodies

The clinical significance of neutralizing antibodies remains controversial, although a higher incidence has been repeatedly observed with IFN-β1b compared with 1a. The PRISMS study reported an inverse dose-dependent effect in the appearance of neutralizing antibodies to IFN-β1a, with some evidence of subsequent effect upon clinical efficacy. This inverse relationship has been reproduced by several trials although without clear effect upon efficacy. The results are confusing, with suggestions of lower development of antibodies at higher doses, but, if present with the higher dose, having a greater impact upon efficacy. Further trials are ongoing in an attempt to determine the significance and long-term effect of these antibodies.

The cost of beta-interferon and glatiramer acetate treatment led to these drugs being early targets for the newly-formed UK National Institute for Clinical Excellence (NICE), whose role includes a cost-effectiveness analysis of new treatments and interventions, to help decide whether treatments are effective and affordable to the UK National Health Service (NHS). Their report from 2002 concluded that these treatments were not cost-effective and should not be used routinely in the NHS in England and Wales, unless costs could be reduced. Not surprisingly, the pharmaceutical industry, together with a vocal patient group, argued strongly against this conclusion, which led to an exploration of alternative ways of spreading the cost and risk of these treatments not being cost effective. The UK 'Risk Sharing Scheme' was essentially developed to enable patient access to treatment at reduced cost, with monitoring of patient disability over time, with the eventual aim of further adjusting prices, depending on data generated by the monitoring scheme. This innovative solution to the NICE report has been criticised, particularly for the lack of scientific rigour of the monitoring scheme, and the missed opportunity for conducting well-designed independent clinical trials rather than simply monitoring patients without a control group. It is now most unlikely that independent long-term clinical trials of these compounds, or any other compounds in which a placebo group is involved, can be conducted in RRMS. Lessons need to be learnt from this saga, and hopefully if more investment in independent clinical trials occurs, linked with a speedier early evaluation of treatments, then similar episodes may be avoided in the future. There is good evidence that patients benefit from taking part in clinical trials, even if receiving placebo treatments. Every opportunity must be taken to obtain high quality scientific data if real disease-modifying treatments are to be identified with confidence.

In the UK, the Association of British Neurologists has produced guidelines on the use of beta-interferon and glatiramer acetate, which are a useful summary of available evidence and recommended practice. These are summarized in Table 15.3 and can be found at http://www.theabn.org/downloads/ABN-MS-Guidelines-2007.pdf

Table 15.2 Summary of effectiveness for beta-interferon

- There is now considerable clinical experience of using these drugs in routine clinical practice.
- Pivotal studies show that these compounds share similar levels of clinical efficacy, although there are two major types of IFN-β (1a and 1b), and three different IFN-β products.
- When used in ambulant patients with RRMS, and a relapse rate of around one per year for the previous 2–3 years (the average relapse rate of RRMS being one every 2 years), patients may expect a reduction in relapses of about 30%.
- Another way of putting this statistic is that if the treatment works and someone is having a relapse a year, over a 3-year period, a patient with RRMS might expect 2 relapses instead of 3.
- The evidence would suggest that these drugs don't work in progressive disease, unless there are concomitant relapses.

Table 15.3 Association of British Neurologists criteria to receive beta-interferon in relapsing-remitting MS

- Able to walk independently, at least 10m with assistance.
- At least 2 clinically significant relapses in the previous 2 years.
- Age 18 or older.
- No contraindications e.g. no monoclonal gammopathy.

Mitoxantrone

Mitoxantrone is a cytotoxic agent licensed for the treatment of leukaemia. It needs to be given intravenously. Original studies used varying doses of mitoxantrone (e.g. $8mg/m^2$ every month for 1 year, or 20mg/month plus methylprednisolone) in differing patient groups (relapsing-remitting, and/or secondary progressive). A total of 93 patients in randomized phase II studies provided evidence that mitoxantrone appeared to be superior to placebo and methylprednisolone in delaying progression and reducing relapse rate.

The principal difficulty in using mitoxantrone is its toxicity, which is probably significantly lower than many other commonly used cytotoxic agents, but limits its use in a chronically disabling condition such as MS, rather than in a lethal illness such as cancer. The two phase II studies failed to demonstrate any significant cardiotoxicity, which has been a major concern with this drug, but confirmed the expected toxic effects of nausea, alopecia, menstrual irregularities, and urinary tract infections.

The pivotal study was a multicentre, placebo controlled, observer blinded, randomized controlled trial comparing low dose ($5mg/m^2$) and high dose ($12mg/m^2$) mitoxantrone with placebo in 194 patients over a 24 month period. Patients had progressive disease, with EDSS scores between 3–6, either with or without relapses, requiring at least one point deterioration in the EDSS score over the previous 18 months to qualify for trial entry. 188 patients were available for assessment at 24 months and the primary outcome was a multivariate analysis of five clinical measures, with significance found in change in EDSS scores, ambulation index, number of treated relapses, time to first treated relapse and change in standardized neurological status. A Cochrane review of 270 patients in clinical trials of mitoxantrone concluded that mitoxantrone reduced the progression of disability and the relapse rate. Although there were no major concerns about safety during the course of these studies, there have subsequently been several cases of acute leukaemia in patients treated with mitoxantrone. The long-term potential cardiotoxicity also requires further evaluation.

Cladribine

Cladribine is a purine nucleoside analogue with particular lymphocyto-toxicity. Previous studies had suggested a beneficial effect in SPMS, with 95% of treated patients stable at one year, supported by favourable MRI parameters. Results from 159 patients with progressive MS (30% PPMS, 70% SPMS), randomized to receive one of two doses of cladribine or placebo by subcutaneous injection for 5 days on a monthly basis for 8 months have been published. Patients were assessed clinically every 2 months, and using MRI every 6 months. The double-blind phase of the study lasted for 12 months. The primary outcome measure was disability, assessed by mean change in EDSS. Mean changes in EDSS did not differ among the groups after 12 months. There was a significant (>90%) reduction in gadolinium-enhancing T1 lesions, largely in the SPMS group. The higher dose of cladribine was found to be relatively safe and also reduced the T2 lesion load slightly. The average patient EDSS at enrolment was 6.0 and the authors report that the trial was underpowered for the patient population enrolled. They also, most probably correctly, report that patients with PPMS may be more resistant to therapy than SPMS, which may well have affected the results. Although 24-month follow-up suggested a trend to beneficial effect in SPMS at both doses, clearly the clinical results from the trial were disappointing. The very sizeable reduction in enhancing lesions, but failure of clinical benefit once again illustrates the discrepancy between MRI and clinical outcomes.

Azathioprine

Azathioprine is a non-specific oral immunosuppressant with a disease modifying action in MS, having a modest benefit both in terms of relapse rate reduction and decreased rate of disease progression. Azathioprine has been used for over 25 years in MS and has never been subject to the sort of rigorous clinical trials used to test beta interferon, although recent small-scale studies seem to show an effect on new MRI lesions, adding to clinical evidence. The immunosuppressive actions of azathioprine are thought to be mediated through 6-mercaptopurine (6-MP) and the production of active thiopurine metabolites, which have both humoral and cell-mediated immunosuppressive effects. It is likely that metabolites released in the conversion of azathioprine to 6-MP are responsible for the hypersensitivity reactions, which often limit its use. Common side effects include skin rash, joint pains, vomiting, and hepatitis. After prolonged use (10–15 years), there is a small increased risk of lymphoma, although risk within the first 10 years of treatment is probably no higher than in the general population. Azathioprine is used more commonly in continental Europe than in North America, with doses gradually increasing according to side effects and lymphocyte counts, but physicians generally aim for around 2–3mg/kg/day. Low levels of the enzyme thiopurine methyl transferase (TPMT) are said to be associated with increased risk of side effects from azathioprine. Recent introduction of enzyme analysis for low levels of TPMT has changed practice in that many people now evaluate TPMT levels before using azathioprine. Some people suggest using lower levels of azathioprine, or not using it at all if enzyme levels are very low. However, some authors also suggest that side effects of azathioprine are not closely linked to TPMT levels. Whilst this area remains controversial, it is recommended that TPMT levels are assessed and caution is used if levels are found to be low.

Pooled immunoglobulins

Immunoglobulins can be extracted from normal human donor blood, and the resulting pooled product can be administered by intravenous infusion to modulate the immune system (IVIg). There are a number of possible modes of action, including inhibition of antibodies, complement, cytokines, and both humoral and cell mediated immunity. In addition, there has been a suggestion from animal studies that IVIg may increase remyelination. The use of IVIg in other inflammatory neurological conditions led initially to several open labelled studies of IVIg in MS, followed by a randomized placebo-controlled trial of monthly IVIg therapy in RRMS (Fazekas et al. 1997). Seventy-five patients with RRMS were randomised to receive IVIg 0.15–0.2g/kg body weight by monthly intravenous infusion for 2 years, (a lower dose than conventionally used in other neurological conditions) and 73 received placebo. Primary outcome measures were an absolute change in EDSS between the two groups (not the conventional method of using EDSS) and the proportion of patients with improved, stable or worse clinical disability, as defined by an increase or decrease of at least one point on the EDSS score, by the end of the study.

Although results were analysed on an intention to treat basis, only 64 IVIg patients and 56 placebo patients completed the trial. The EDSS score, decreased in the IVIg patients (−0.23) and increased in the placebo patients (0.12, $p = 0.008$) and there was also a significant difference in the number of relapses between the 2 groups: 116 in the placebo group and 62 in the IVIg group over the study period (reduction of 59%). Subsequent analysis suggested that the reduction in disability in the IVIg treated group was obtained in the first 6 months of the study, and disability remained fairly constant thereafter. The reduction in relapse rate, however, was seen throughout the study period. The authors suggest that this may be due to early remyelination, enhanced by IVIg, whereas the immunmodulatory action of the drug may persist throughout the period of its use. Unfortunately there was no MRI analysis in this study, and there were concerns raised over investigator blinding.

A Cochrane review and meta-analysis of further IVIg studies in MS have concluded that there may be a role for IVIg in treatment of relapses in RRMS, but the lack of robust evidence using conventional progression measures is a problem, as is the relative paucity of MRI evidence.

The dose of IVIg in the original studies was chosen to be lower than is normally used for inflammatory neuromuscular conditions, in order to reduce potential complications, which include anaphylaxis, acute renal failure, cerebral thrombosis, and transmission of infections. Although IVIg undergoes rigorous production methods in order to minimize the potential infectious risk, the concern that hitherto undiscovered infectious agents could be transmitted by these infusions cannot be discounted.

More recently the European Study on Immunoglobulin in MS (ESIMS) has been reported. This is a 318 patient study of IVIg (1g/kg body weight by monthly infusion versus placebo) in SPMS. There was no effect on the primary outcome measure of confirmed sustained deterioration in EDSS, or in relapse rate, time to deterioration in EDSS, or most of the MRI parameters. There is therefore no evidence to support the use of IVIg in progressive MS, arguing against a possible role for IVIg in enhancing remyelination. The overall evidence for the use of IVIg in MS is therefore rather weak.

Methotrexate

Methotrexate resembles folic acid and competes with it for dihydrofolate reductase, thereby preventing the synthesis of nuclear material and ultimately leading to cell death. It may also have independent effects on immunoregulation and an anti-inflammatory action (for example it may reduce interleukin-1 action by binding it, as there is a 60% sequence homology between IL-1b and dihydrofolate reductase). It is tolerated better than azathioprine or cyclophosphamide and is usually given orally once a week.

In a small randomized placebo-controlled double-blind study of 20 RRMS and 24 SPMS patients given 7.5mg methotrexate/week and followed up for 18 months, there appeared to be a marginal reduction in relapse rate in the RRMS group, but no significant change in EDSS over this period and no effect in chronic progressive patients (Currier *et al.* 1993).

Similar doses of methotrexate were used in a further randomized double-blind placebo-controlled study in 60 patients with chronic progressive MS over a 2 year period (Goodkin *et al.* 1995). Treatment failure (and hence disease progression) was defined in a number of ways according to deterioration for more than 2 months in any one of the four assessment measures: EDSS reduction by 0.5–1.0 points (depending on initial EDSS score), ambulation index reduction by one point, or 20% reduction in timed performance in a box and block test or 9-hole peg test. Overall, 51.6% of the group taking methotrexate deteriorated according to one of these measures, compared with 82.8% of the placebo group. However, there was no difference in EDSS and ambulation index scores, or box and block test times, between the two groups, and the only significant effect appeared to be in 9-hole peg testing. Interestingly, at the end of the study, patients, doctors and nurses were asked to give a 'global impression' of whether the treatment had made any difference to the patients: no significant effect of treatment was found. There was no significant difference in the level of side effects between methotrexate and placebo groups, confirming its tolerability.

Although higher doses of methotrexate have been tested in people with MS, as yet there is no convincing evidence to support the routine use of high dose methotrexate.

Cyclosporin

Cyclosporin was originally isolated from fungi and was found to have immunosuppressive activity, being of particular use in preventing organ rejection after transplantation. Its use is associated with a high incidence of side effects including nephrotoxicity and hypertension. It may have a marginal effect in progressive disease, with trials showing a small but significant change in EDSS scores and in the time to becoming wheelchair bound. It is a difficult drug to use, as blood levels are required to adjust doses, and most people would accept that any minimal benefit is outweighed by the side-effect profile.

Cyclophosphamide

This potent alkylating agent, which kills all actively dividing cells and hence causes a dose-dependent bone marrow suppression, has been used in progressive MS for a number of years. Initial studies seemed to suggest an effect in stabilizing progressive MS, but at the expense of significant side effects. Although no infections were reported in the IV cyclophosphamide-treated groups, all patients lost their hair, 30% experienced nausea, some patients experienced microscopic haematuria, and peripheral blood white cell counts dropped an average of 89%.

Interpretation of the studies is difficult, as the most significant factor involved in producing these apparently beneficial effects was the poor clinical course of the control group, who showed significantly lower stabilization than both natural history data and data from placebo groups in other trials. Although this research team subsequently reported an 81% stabilization in 164 openly treated patients over a 6 year period (Carter *et al.* 1988), the only other large-scale placebo-controlled single-masked study (the Canadian Cooperative Multiple Sclerosis Study Group Trial, 1991) failed to show any significant treatment effect when compared to placebo. In this study 55 patients were randomized to receive IV cyclophosphamide and oral prednisolone, 57 received oral cyclophosphamide, oral prednisolone and weekly plasma exchange, and 56 patients received placebo medications and sham plasma exchange. Attempts were made to blind the examining clinician by bandaging all patients' heads and arms to mask any allopecia or evidence of plasma exchange. All patients were followed up for at least 12 months (mean 30.4 months) and no significant differences were demonstrated in the EDSS scores in any 6-month period over the course of the study. Although cyclophosphamide still has its proponents, most people would accept that any evidence of benefit is outweighed by potential side effects, and more potent drugs have superseded it.

Alemtuzumab (Campath® 1H)

Scientific progress in the creation of antibodies in the late twentieth century was associated with other technological advances; antibodies could be created in rodents so that the fragment of the antibody binding to the antigen is rat derived, but the rest of the antibody molecule is human (so-called humanized monoclonal antibodies). This has the advantage of generating less of an immune response against the antibody molecule itself when used therapeutically.

Alemtuzumab is a humanized monoclonal antibody against CD52, a cell surface antigen on lymphocytes and monocytes. It was first created in Cambridge in the 1980s, and used therapeutically in MS since then. Most of the published evidence is from open label use, which is impressive. There is a dramatic effect both on MRI activity but also episodes of clinical relapse. Experience demonstrated most effect on aggressive MS early on in the disease course. In fact most immunomodulatory treatments used in progressive forms of MS, have demonstrated that any marginal effects in progressive patients are probably outweighed by side effects. Early excitement in alemtuzumab use was eventually followed by a multicentre randomized trial comparing high dose beta-interferon with alemtuzumab, as a placebo arm was considered unethical. Unfortunately, there was an unexpected death from the treatable condition autoimmune thrombocytopenia. An interim analysis has confirmed exciting positive benefits, with significant improvements in relapse rate in the alemtuzumab arm of the study, with >75% reduction in relapse rate compared to high dose IFN-β (Rebif®), together with seemingly solid data on disease progression. However, the occurrence of thrombocytopenia was confirmed in more cases, and the incidence of other autoimmune diseases was also confirmed. It was known before the study commenced that up to 30% of cases might develop thyrotoxicosis following alemtuzumab treatment, with rare dysthyroid eye disease. There has also been a case of autoimmune renal disease. This drug therefore seems to be very effective at switching MS off (at least temporarily), but can unearth other autoimmune tendencies, even though the vast majority of these are easily treatable. It is likely that careful monitoring will still mean that the risk/benefit ratio in this case will be swayed more to the benefit side. The drug may therefore have a significant role in stabilizing aggressive disease and appears to be the most promising of the emerging therapies. Phase III studies are now underway, but as the drug already has a license for treating chronic lymphatic leukaemia, and it is considerably cheaper than some alternatives, it is being used in carefully selected patients in some MS centres.

Alemtuzumab is currently given intravenously on a daily basis, initially for 5 days, and then again after 12 months. Further doses may also be appropriate, possibly after longer intervals. Because the drug causes massive cell death of lymphocytes, a release of cytokines can occur acutely, which can reduce nerve conduction in previously demyelinated pathways. To prevent this temporary reaction, intravenous steroids are administered an hour before the alemtuzumab. Otherwise acute administration is often associated with an allergic type rash, best treated with antihistamines. If used, regular blood tests for blood count, renal and thyroid function and autoantibody evaluation are mandatory.

Natalizumab (Antegren®, Tysabri®)

Natalizumab (NZB) is a humanized monoclonal antibody to α4 integrin, an adhesion molecule involved in the traffic of lymphocytes across the blood-brain barrier, which interacts with endothelial adhesion molecules including vascular cell adhesion molecule-1 (VCAM-1). It is administered intravenously, and has been used in the treatment of Crohn's disease and RRMS. Initial studies using various dosing frequencies showed possible clinical effect, largely based on results from MRI studies. The decision was made to proceed to phase 3 studies. Two recent trials have been conducted. Both recruited patients who had experienced at least one relapse in the previous year, each comparing the annualised relapse rate at one year as the primary end point. The AFFIRM study randomized patients in a 2:1 ration to NZB or placebo, and the SENTINEL study recruited over 500 patients in each arm who had experienced at least one relapse despite treatment with IFN-β1a (Avonex®), with one arm being Avonex® and placebo infusions, and the other being Avonex® and NZB.

Results from a planned one year analysis of effect on relapse rate seemed to demonstrate a substantial effect. On the basis of these unpublished data, with median safety data exposure of 20 months, NZB was fast-tracked by the US Food and Drug Administration to obtain a license for treating RRMS. Subsequent to the granting of a license, it emerged that 3 patients had developed progressive multifocal leucoencephalopathy (PML), a progressive, usually fatal, viral infection in immunocompromised individuals, most commonly seen in AIDS. In fact, one of these patients had been exposed to NZB in relation to Crohn's disease, and was thought to have died with a brain tumour, but this diagnosis was subsequently revised after two MS patients developed PML. One of these patients died (who turned out not to have the expected changes of MS at autopsy), and the other survived with severe disabilities. As a result of these cases of PML, the drug was withdrawn.

The final results from both of these studies were published in 2006 and confirmed large apparent effects in relapse rate reduction. After one year, in AFFIRM, there was a reduction from 0.81 relapses/year in the placebo group, to 0.26 in the NZB group (a 68% relative rate reduction). In SENTINEL, the rates were 0.82 relapses/year in beta-interferon alone, to 0.38 in the NZB group (a 54% reduction).

After 2 years, the proportion of people who had progressed to 'sustained disability' at 3 monthly intervals in AFFIRM was 29% in the placebo group and 17% in the NZB group (42% decrease). In SENTINEL this was 29% with beta-interferon alone, and 23% with NZB (24% decrease). These figures all reached statistical significance. If we look at the more useful 6 monthly sustained disability criterion, then there was still a statistically significant 54% reduction sustained disability in the AFFIRM study, but no significant effect in SENTINEL (18% progression with interferon alone and 15% in combination group).

As in many studies, the effect on MRI was very dramatic in both studies, with 92% less enhancing lesions in the active arm of the AFFIRM study and 89% in SENTINEL. We must always remember that we are treating people and not MR scans, but the MR results are encouraging and provide support to the clinical relapse data to suggest that levels of inflammation are substantially reduced with NZB over the 2-year treatment period.

This episode has generated considerable debate, not least the wisdom of licensing a drug based on short-term data via a fast-track, non-published, or peer-reviewed route. On the other hand, the initial clinical results seemed promising and, if taken with the more exciting alemtuzumab data, might suggest that in more aggressive disease, patients and clinicians might have the option of trying aggressive chemotherapy, in the knowledge of potential serious side effects. The difficulty is in identifying those individuals who are more likely to benefit from treatments with higher degrees of risk, so that the risk/benefit decision is worth taking.

This difficult risk-benefit equation was taken into account when the drug was re-introduced into clinical use in mid-2006. Although the trials involved people with MS who had had at least one relapse in the previous year, the licensed indications are somewhat different. This is related to the risk of PML, so that in order to justify the risk/benefit ratio, only people with severe disease or having failed on beta-interferon are recommended at the moment. Specifically:

- Patients with high disease activity despite treatment with a beta-interferon, with at least one relapse in the previous year while on therapy and at least 9 T2 lesions on cranial MRI, or at least one gadolinium enhancing lesion.
- Patients with rapidly evolving severe relapsing remitting MS, defined by 2 or more disabling relapses in one year, and one or more gadolinium enhancing lesion on brain MR, or significant increase in T2 lesions compared to previous MRI.

Clearly these criteria are much more stringent than the original trials. This begs the question of whether there is any evidence that this more severe group of patients will actually respond to treatment. There has been some evaluation of the more severely affected patients in the two studies. It is always frowned upon to perform retrospective subgroup analysis in studies that were not designed to address the question being asked. However, if the licensed criteria are applied, then the relapse rate in the NZB group is 0.282 (n = 148) compared to 1.455 (n = 61) in the placebo group (data from manufacturers' summary of product characteristics).

One of the other major considerations around the use of NZB is its cost, which in the UK is around twice the price of interferon, and, if monitoring costs are taken into account, may turn out to be nearer three times the price. At the time of writing, this drug is being evaluated by NICE in cost-effectiveness terms.

Treatments for progressive disease

Unfortunately there is no good evidence for any drug having an effect in progressive forms of MS in the absence of relapses. Many clinicians, often after heartfelt discussion with patients, have tried powerful immunotherapies at this stage of the illness, but with little, if any, success. This is compatible with the hypothesis that if immunotherapies are going to work, they must be used early in the illness. There is mounting evidence from natural history studies that once walking starts to become affected in people with MS, then there is a steady decline in physical functioning, which at present cannot be halted. A degree of optimism can be given to patients by telling them that the majority of people with MS will not die from their disease, and disability does tend to stabilize over time, but it is impossible to predict at what point that will occur, or how disabled people will be when things settle down.

Treatment of relapses

Comprehensive multidisciplinary management of relapse

An acute relapse refers to an episode of neurological disturbance that lasts for at least 24 hours, and for which there is no other cause such as fever. Typically a relapse evolves over a few days, reaches a plateau, and then remits to a variable degree over a few weeks or months (refer to Chapter 4) . The patient experiencing a relapse has to cope with a comparatively sudden onset of neurological symptoms that may be physically and psychologically distressing and functionally and socially incapacitating. In the longer term, incomplete remission from a relapse may result in residual neurological deficit. Management of an acute relapse requires a comprehensive approach addressing its medical, functional, and psychosocial effects. Management incorporates education regarding relapses, support in the event of a relapse, treatment to accelerate or improve the recovery from a relapse, and symptomatic treatment and rehabilitation.

In terms of relapses, people should be given information regarding general health factors, such as infection, which may influence the risk of relapse, advised on how to detect relapses, and what to do if new symptoms occur, including how to self-refer into primary or secondary care clinics.

In the event of new or increased symptoms people with MS should be able to identify and contact a professional from their healthcare team who can advise them or direct them to the most appropriate local service. If a person with MS develops new or increased neurological symptoms a formal assessment should be made to determine the diagnosis. At the assessment the possibility of any other medical cause for an increase in neurological symptoms must be considered. In particular it is important to exclude an infective cause such as a urinary tract infection, which may be otherwise clinically silent. The possibility of dual neurological pathology, for example, a cord compression mimicking a spinal cord relapse, should also be borne in mind. If the new symptoms are assessed to be unrelated to MS it must still be ensured that the person with MS has access to the appropriate service and treatment.

Management of acute relapses should not just be limited to corticosteroid therapy but should be comprehensive, tackling all aspects of the relapse. Practical supportive measures, such as the provision of care or equipment, may be essential and should not be forgotten. Symptomatic treatment for new symptoms from a relapse may sometimes be required. If a relapse is improving spontaneously or with corticosteroids the duration of symptoms may be too short to warrant symptomatic treatment. However, if symptoms are distressing or not resolving then treatment may be required. Symptomatic treatments are not discussed further here but are covered in Chapter 26.

Functional recovery from a relapse may be facilitated by multidisciplinary input from neurological rehabilitation services. This input should run in collaboration with any medical treatment and depending on need may be on anoutpatient or inpatient basis. There is evidence that a multidisciplinary rehabilitation approach is superior to a standard ward routine in people with MS receiving intravenous corticosteroid therapy. Inpatient rehabilitation has also been shown to be useful in RRMS particularly in people with incomplete recovery from relapses with moderate to severe disability.

Protocol for treatment of MS relapses

A protocol for the medical management of MS relapse is given in Table 16.1.

Table 16.1

A **relapse** in multiple sclerosis is the onset of new or worsening neurological symptoms of greater than 24 hour duration. Most relapses do not require hospitalization and many patients tolerate mild deterioration in their condition without seeking medical attention. The patient is usually the best person to tell us how bad the relapse is, and therefore whether it should be treated with steroids.It is important to differentiate a relapse from a pseudo-relapse, which is a temporary worsening of pre-existing symptoms due to concurrent fever, illness, or infection. Pseudo-relapses never present with new symptoms, often lasting only a few hours, and their treatment should be directed towards the precipitating cause.

1) History of deterioration
- Are these new symptoms, worsening of present symptoms, or recurrence of old symptoms?—Relapses can present with any of these, but new symptoms are more suggestive of definite relapse.
- When did this episode of deterioration start?
- Are symptoms stable, still deteriorating, or improving?—If starting to improve then consider a watch and wait policy.
- Any recent infection which may have precipitated relapse?

N.B. Multiple episodes of paroxysmal symptoms such as tonic spasms or trigeminal neuralgia occurring over not less than 24 hours may also constitute a relapse.

2) MS history
- Date of diagnosis.
- MS phenotype (RRMS, SPMS, PPMS).
- Number of relapses requiring steroids over the previous 2 years—this is important in considering other long-term treatment options.

3) Examination
- Temperature, pulse, and blood pressure.
- Pharyngeal examination for erythema or pus.
- Chest auscultation.
- Detailed neurological examination including visual acuity.

4) Investigations
- Dipstick urinalysis; MSU to lab.
- Throat swab in cases of suspected pharyngitis.
- Sputum culture if productive cough.
- Blood cultures if T ≥100°F.

Table 16.1 (*Contd.*)

5) Treatment for confirmed relapses
Either:

a) Intravenous methylprednisolone 1g in 100ml normal saline daily over 30min for 3 consecutive days. This can be organized as inpatient (especially if severe relapse requiring physiotherapy etc.), as a day case, or in local GP surgeries or other hospitals or at home if facilities are available.

Or:

b) Oral methylprednisolone 500mg daily for 5 consecutive days after a meal. This method is often preferred as people don't need to stay in hospital. A formal trial comparison of oral versus IV has not been performed in large numbers of people.

• There is no evidence that oral tail of steroids is superior to short courses.

• If patient has a history of gastric ulcers or gastric irritation with previous courses of steroids, cover with omeprazole 20mg daily.

• Advise the patient about the possible side effects of steroids: metallic taste in the mouth, facial flushing, insomnia, stomach upset, restlessness, mood swings, often mild euphoria, rarely psychosis or depression.

6) Others

• Consider other needs of the patient, refer to physiotherapy and/or OT services as required.

• If more than 2 relapses have occurred in the last 2 years refer to MS clinic for consideration of disease-modifying therapy.

Chapter 17

Other treatments available

Hyperbaric oxygen

Treatments for MS frequently go through a phase of optimistic fervour generally spread by word of mouth or the internet. Often interest in treatments, and a demand for their availability, precedes any evidence for efficacy. Unfortunately, the list of unsuccessful treatments far exceeds the list of useful ones. Hyperbaric oxygen therapy is one such treatment. Many oxygen chambers are still in existence and used to treat MS, although there is no evidence of any efficacy, and indeed this is an example of a treatment where there is definite evidence for lack of efficacy. A Cochrane review and several other authors reach similar conclusions.

Bee venom

Venom from the honeybee contains substances with anti-inflammatory properties and may inhibit calcium activated potassium channels. This treatment has increased in popularity and until recently there had been no evidence on which to make any rational decisions. A recent randomized crossover study of live bee exposure (up to 20 bees 3 times per week) failed to demonstrate any beneficial effect on cranial MRI or any clinical parameters. Not surprisingly, quality of life was also not improved!

Goat serum

This treatment has recently gone through a phase of popularity in the UK, without any evidence for efficacy. This substance is produced by immunizing goats with an undisclosed human protein, and then isolating the goat serum for injection. The rationale for using this treatment is rather obscure, and recent studies within the UK were either negative or not completed. It is possible to obtain this substance privately, suggesting that financial motives may dominate. There is no evidence that this drug has any therapeutic value in any condition and people with MS should be discouraged from considering it.

Low dose naltrexone

This is another therapy with no evidence for efficacy, but in which there has been some recent interest. Naltrexone is an opiate antagonist, and doses of around 50mg are usually needed to produce pharmacological action at opiate receptors. There have been anecdotal reports of low doses (around 2.5mg) having an effect in limited clinical situations, the apparent theory being that low doses may stimulate the immune system and therefore benefit people with MS (a rationale running contrary to most scientific evidence). It remains to be seen whether a clinical trial will emerge in this area.

Stem cells

This area of potential treatment has generated considerable excitement, both in the scientific community and among patients. It is important to consider exact terminology, as not all stem cells are the same. The term stem cell refers to a precursor cell type that can both self-renew and differentiate down particular pathways to generate some or all tissues of the body. They can be classified into a number of categories, including:

- Embryonic stem cells—from fertilized eggs or embryos, usually at the blastocyst stage of development. These are believed to be capable of developing into all cell types. This type of cell is the focus of intense research activity, particularly by investigators using genetic cloning techniques, so that instead of requiring normal human embryos, it might be possible to clone these cells in the laboratory by genetic manipulation.
- Pluripotent progenitor cells—from embryos, foetus or neonate, that are already partially committed to differentiate down a particular pathway (e.g. neurons). This group includes multipotent neuroepithelial stem cells and lineage restricted neuronal precursors. Such cells have also been found in the adult paraventricular zone in the central nervous system, countering the long-held views that the mammalian nervous system has no innate capacity for regeneration.
- Mesenchymal stem cells—usually derived from bone marrow. This type of stem cell is commonly used in bone marrow transplantation for treating haematological malignancies. Under these circumstances, cells are usually mobilized from the bone marrow into the peripheral blood for harvesting before reinjection. Earlier forms of stem cell may be available if bone marrow is harvested directly by biopsy, and this type of cell may be more useful for treating MS.
- Other stem cells, including umbilical cord stem cells.

All of these stem cell types have been suggested as possible sources of cells for the treatment of MS. However, at the time of writing, these approaches remain entirely experimental. There is no evidence that any human being has benefited from stem cell transplantation for the treatment of MS. All kinds of problems need to be overcome, including an understanding of the control mechanisms in proliferation and differentiation, so that the theoretical risk of tumour formation is avoided. Another problem with any transplantation of non-self tissue, is the potential for stimulating an immune response to the transplanted cell. This is avoided if autologous (self) tissue, such as own bone marrow stem cells, is used. Once again, any new potential treatment is open to exploitation by medical practitioners wishing to cash in on high patient expectation and desperation. Some people are paying large amounts of money to travel for untested treatments in the hope that a cure may be achieved. Whilst this course of action is entirely understandable, in the present state of scientific knowledge these people are likely to be disappointed and at worst, may be exposing themselves to considerable risk.

Cannabis and cannabinoids

The cannabis plant is a source of many useful substances. Most of its therapeutic potential is thought to lie in the more than 60 different cannabinoids present in the plant. The most active of these is Δ^9tetra-hydrocannabinol (Δ^9THC or dronabinol). Word of mouth reporting of beneficial effects of smoked cannabis on MS symptoms, including pain, urinary disturbance, tremor, and particularly spasticity, led to newspaper reports and anecdotal accounts being published in the medical literature. This caused widespread unlicensed and often illegal use of cannabinoids in MS, via a number of varying formulations and routes of administration. These range from smoked cannabis leaf to oral preparations including cannabis oil, extracted cannabinoids, and synthetic cannabinoids such as Nabilone. The MS Society estimates that between 1 and 4% of the total MS population in the UK is illegally using cannabis for relief of symptoms (up to 2750 patients).

Most cannabinoid effects appear to be mediated through cannabinoid receptors, two types of which have been isolated and cloned: CB_1 and CB_2. CB_1 receptors are distributed widely in the nervous system, and seem to have a general role in the inhibition of neurotransmitter release, whereas CB_2 receptors are principally found on cells of the immune system. The discovery of a range of endogenous endocannabinoids, the most important of which are thought to be 2-arachidonoylglycerol (2-AG) and arachidonoylethanolamide (anandamide), has also provoked considerable interest. The experimental basis behind a neuroprotective action for cannabinoids is becoming more convincing, with neuroprotective effects having been demonstrated in animal models of head injury and multiple sclerosis. There is also laboratory evidence showing cannabinoids reduce glutamate release and calcium flux as well as being antioxidants, thereby reducing free radical damage. Excess excitatory neurotransmitter (especially glutamate) release, increased calcium influx, and free radical damage, have all been implicated in neuronal death, and treatment strategies in neurodegenerative conditions have focused on reducing the impact of some or all of these mechanisms. In addition, CB_1 receptor activation has been shown to reduce oligodendrocyte apoptosis in vitro, which may be of significance to some progressive forms of MS.

The recent Cannabinoids in MS (CAMS) study focused on testing symptomatic benefits from cannabinoids over a 15-week period, and is the largest of a number of recent studies in this area. Participants are included on the basis of having relatively stable MS in the 6 months prior to study recruitment, and were randomized to receive oral cannabis extract, dronabinol, or placebo capsules. Of the 630 who received treatment, 95% had progressive disease. Following the main 15-week trial period, patients were offered the opportunity to continue medication in a blinded fashion for up to 12 months, during which period both disability measures and symptomatic assessments were performed. The primary outcome measure assessed spasticity using the best available measurement at the time—the Ashworth scale. No treatment effect on spasticity was found during the main study, although patients felt active medication was much more helpful than placebo in alleviating some of their distressing symptoms. This may partly demonstrate the relative insensitivity of the Ashworth scale and certainly suggests that spasticity is a very complex phenomenon. During the course of the study, experimental evidence was emerging to suggest that cannabinoids might have a neuroprotective action, which led to particular interest in the results of the 12-month follow-up study. The results of the follow-up study showed significant effects on spasticity scores in the dronabinol arm, but not the cannabis extract arm. There is also some evidence for an effect on disability, measured by the Expanded Disability Status Scale (EDSS) and the Rivermead Mobility Index. It is worth stressing that although the effect size in the follow-up study was modest, the investigators had not expected to see any effect over a relatively short follow-up period in this group of very disabled but relatively stable patients. The CAMS follow-up results provide the first clinical evidence to support increasing experimental data raising the possibility of a neuroprotective effect of cannabinoids, as well as confirming that these medicines continued to ameliorate patient symptoms. A new long-term study is now being conducted over a 3-year period, to investigate possible effects of dronabinol on disease progression. This is known as the Cannabinoid Use in Progressive Inflammatory brain Disease (CUPID) study.

Other studies of cannabinoids have either taken place, or are in the process of being conducted. One of the major problems in this area is in providing convincing data that patient-reported symptoms respond to treatment, and are not simply due to a non-specific benefit, possibly resulting from unblinding and potential bias due to the side effects of active medication. Other methods of administering cannabinoids are also being explored including an oromucosal spray (Sativex®).

Drugs in development

There are currently around 150 treatments under evaluation in MS. The majority of these target specific aspects of the immune system, including passage of cells across the blood-brain barrier, all components of the immunological synapse (between T-cell and antigen presenting cell, see Chapter 3), cytokines and other communication molecules, as well as methods of reducing immune cell activation. In addition, some treatments are being tested in progressive disease, where neuronal death is thought to substantially explain the gradual accumulation of disability. Such treatments include drugs to block excess calcium release, excess sodium channel activation (e.g. lamotrigine), free radical damage, damage secondary to abnormal respiration, blockers of excitatory neurotransmitters, and also growth factors to enhance cell survival.

Other experimental approaches include investigating ways of encouraging neuronal regeneration (such as by blocking inhibitors of axon growth), preventing scar formation, and encouraging other ways of promoting neuronal plasticity.

Diet

Many people with MS are concerned about the impact of MS on lifestyle and are interested in finding out about the role of diet in maintenance of health. There is no substantial evidence to support special diets such as gluten free; however, many people incorporate such diets into their self-management plans. People often ask if alcohol is contraindicated. There is no evidence that moderate intake of alcohol affects MS disease activity although it may impact on urinary symptoms (it is a bladder irritant), or exacerbate balance, mobility or speech problems. It is advisable to check if alcohol is contraindicated with some prescribed medications and should be avoided when receiving steroid treatment or using non-steroidal anti-inflammatory medications. A minimum daily intake of 1.5 litres of water is advised for maintenance of health.

The role of essential fatty acids in MS has been researched with some evidence suggesting that omega 6 linoelic acid may be of benefit. Although there is still some debate about the exact role of essential fatty acids in MS there is agreement that linoelic acid is an important element of a healthy diet. In the UK, NICE Guidelines advise that an intake of 17–23g per day of linoleic acid may slow down the disabling effects of MS.

Overall, in the absence of allergy and intolerance, people with MS should be advised that a diet balanced with low saturated fats, carbohydrates and 'five a day' fruit or vegetables is recommended. People should be made aware that the occasional treat that is high in saturated fat, sugar or salt will not cause harm and that a well balanced diet should cover all nutritional requirements, without need for nutritional supplements.

People with MS who are over or underweight or have symptoms that interfere with feeding or swallowing should be referred to appropriate team members including dieticians, speech and language therapists, nurses, and occupational therapists for advice and support to optimize dietary and fluid intake.

Part 4

Ongoing management

Principles of ongoing management

Introduction

The multiplicity of symptoms that may arise as a result of MS means that the physical, cognitive and psychosocial consequences are often wide-ranging, variable and complex. Because the disease evolves at differing rates over several decades, the needs of the individual will change over time, often quite suddenly and unexpectedly. These needs extend from the core medical parameters, and may include every facet of individual, family and community existence. Effective overall management of the individual therefore involves taking a long-term and proactive approach to management which begins from the point of diagnosis and continues throughout their lifetime. It requires an approach which acknowledges that this life-long disease requires a continuing relationship to be developed wherein the person with MS needs to be able to access services in a timely manner, as their needs change. Unfortunately surveys demonstrate that this contrasts starkly with the reality for many people whose experience of health and social care service input is overwhelmingly one of crises management wherein interventions are provided as a fragmented series of short term quick fixes.

Adopting a rehabilitation approach

Rehabilitation should not be viewed as a particular component of health care for people with MS. Rather, the person and all those involved in their care should be encouraged to adopt a 'rehabilitation approach' to the ongoing management of their condition, at every stage of the condition from initial diagnosis.

Rehabilitation has been defined as '... an active process of change by which a person who has become disabled acquires and uses the knowledge and skill necessary for optimal physical, psychological and social function'[1]. A key underlying principle of rehabilitation is that the affected person and their family become central to planning and participating in their own management programme, in order to ensure interventions remain relevant to their own changing needs and circumstances. This is achieved through an ongoing process of education wherein the maintenance of activities is emphasized (despite the presence of symptoms and limitations) by equipping the person with effective coping skills so that they can manage deficits and apply solutions to challenges. By promoting physical, psychological and social adaptation, the aim of adopting a rehabilitation approach to management is to improve the quality of life of all those affected by the disease. This is viewed as a constantly evolving and ongoing process which is relevant and applicable at every stage of the condition from initial diagnosis to those with severe disability.

Incorporating this approach into ongoing care

In considering the needs of people with MS and how a rehabilitation approach should be incorporated throughout the course of the disease, it is helpful to divide the condition into four stages:

- Diagnosis
- Minimal disability
- Moderate disability
- Severe disability.

A practical framework for considering the key needs and main focus of care at each of these stages is presented in Table 18.1.

There are consistent themes running through each of these stages which include:

- Access to up-to-date information
- Appropriate expertise, often of a multi-disciplinary nature
- Flexibility and accessibility
- Good communication
- Empowerment of the person with MS

Adoption of a rehabilitation approach to management is central to successfully meeting these needs throughout the continuum of the disease.

---

1 Disability Committee of the Royal College of Physicians, 1981 London, HMSO.

Table 18.1 A practical framework for considering the key needs and main focus of care at different stages of MS

Phase of MS	Key needs	Main focus of care
Diagnostic phase	• Certain, clear diagnosis • Appropriate support at diagnosis • The provision of disease-modifying drugs as appropriate • Access to information • Continuing education	The main focus should be on self-management with an emphasis on the concept of wellness, incorporating diet, exercise, and a healthy lifestyle.
Minimal disability	• Advice, support and information • Self-management options • Treatment of relapses including disease-modifying agents • Treatment of other conditions	The main focus of care should be on self-management, with input from members of the multidisciplinary team as required
Moderate disability	• Rehabilitation and symptomatic management • Easy access to responsive and coordinated services • Appropriate level of expertise • Good communication • Self-management	A comprehensive rehabilitation programme may be particularly appropriate at this stage
Severe disability	• Access to information and expertise • Good communication and co-ordinated care • Adequate community care services • Flexible provision of respite care	Appropriate long-term care provision including palliative care

After, Freeman JA, Ford H, Mattison P, et al. *Developing MS Healthcare Standards: evidence-based recommendations for service providers.* Multiple Sclerosis Society of Great Britain and Northern Ireland. March 2002.

Guided self-management

People with MS have an important role to play, not only in forming a partnership with professionals in terms of making decisions, but also in actively managing their own care and management. They should be encouraged and allowed to assume responsibility for maintaining the best possible health status. This approach is often referred to as self-management. Fundamental to the concept of self-management is that the person is able to make an informed judgement about their own decisions. Some basic tenets in patient motivation should be acknowledged in promoting self-management (Table 18.2)

Education about the disease and its management is essential to facilitate self-management. This education should not simply be in the form of pre-printed, standardized information leaflets and self-management plans but should involve a process wherein the individual is helped to work out when, why and how things go astray. The rationale underlying this is that the person's improved understanding of the nature of their symptoms and reasons for the treatment approach enables better control of symptoms, and a clearer idea of when they should seek help. Effective long term management of a whole array of common symptoms such as spasticity, fatigue and incontinence ultimately relies on the success of this approach. This should begin early in the disease course so that common, often preventable complications such as de-conditioning, disuse weakness and muscle shortening, can be minimized, and quality of life optimized.

There are a number of key requirements and core skills needed to self-manage a disease. These are summarized in Tables 18.3 and 18.4 respectively.

It should be recognized that there are a number of challenges to self-management in MS. These include:

- The presence of cognitive impairments such as impairments of memory, concentration, lack of insight, and other cognitive capacities.
- Reduced motivation of the individual and/or their family.
- Lack of self-confidence to undertake the task, and to self-advocate. It should be recognized that while some patients can be successful at self-advocacy, many are not.
- Inaccurate information, for example some of the information freely accessible on the internet.
- Lack of knowledge about the potential problems and possible solutions, including when to self-refer to health or social service professionals for further help.
- 'Don't wish to worry the doctors' syndrome.
- Lack of access to services.

All of these factors can impact markedly on the ability of the person to make informed decisions and to effectively self-manage. It is therefore important that when problems arise, the person with MS can have access to assessment by a professional or team of professionals. This can enable the nature of the problem to be established and a plan of management, which is decided in partnership with the individual to be instigated.

Table 18.2 Basic tenets in patient motivation

Patients are more likely to seek and actively participate in appropriate interventions if a number of key factors are considered and addressed:

1. Knowledge of the basic nature and prognosis of MS (including natural history of the disease, major clinical manifestations, nature of relapses, other causes of fluctuating symptoms).
2. Information about treatments and their effects.
3. Involvement in decisions about treatment.
4. Good communication with professionals involved in their care.
5. Prompt and effective support when problems occur.
6. Ongoing monitoring of progress.

Table 18.3 Requirements to self-manage a chronic disease:

- Knowing how to recognize and act upon symptoms.
- Dealing with acute attacks of disease.
- Making effective use of treatments/medicines.
- Comprehending the implications of professional advice.
- Establishing a sleep pattern and dealing with fatigue.
- Managing work.
- Accessing leisure activities.
- Developing strategies to deal with the psychological impact of the disease.
- Learning to cope with other people's response to your illness.

After Department of Health (2001) The expert patient: a new approach to chronic disease management for the 21st century. Department of Health 2001. Available at: http://www.dh.gov.uk

Table 18.4 Five core self-management skills in managing a chronic disease:

- Problem solving
- Decision making
- Resource utilization
- Forming patient/health professional partnership
- Taking action.

After Department of Health (2001) The expert patient: a new approach to chronic disease management for the 21st century. Department of Health 2001. Available at: http://www.dh.gov.uk

Rehabilitation strategies such as goal setting and problem solving are also useful in guiding self-management and assisting the professional in developing a sustained working relationship with individuals. This partnership must extend beyond the person with MS to include carers and family members, particularly when cognitive and physical difficulties mean that the person becomes more heavily reliant on others for self-care and making decisions related to their daily life.

There are a wide range of resources available which the patient can use to improve their self management skills. These include:

- The Expert Patient Programme—which helps people to seek, evaluate, and use advice and help available; to manage common symptoms; and to communicate effectively with healthcare professionals. These courses take place over 6 weeks and are led by people who, themselves, live with a long-term medical condition (further information available at *http://www.expertpatients.nhs.uk*)
- Local and national MS support organizations, which provide information packs and educational programmes to cover all aspects of MS. They also host internet based discussion forums and provide telephone support to assist with a whole range of issues relating to self-management (refer to Chapter 32 on useful websites and resources).
- Local courses, usually coordinated by specialist MS nurses, which are aimed at providing a range of information about MS and details of local support available. Typically these are aimed at the person who is newly diagnosed.

Education is not a one-way street. While the need for education of the person with MS has been stressed, it cannot be overemphasized how important it is for professionals to acknowledge the expertise of people with MS. This is particularly the case for people who have lived with their disability for a long time and who may be considered 'experts' as to their own specific needs.

Active involvement of the individual in treatment decisions

Most people with MS want to be involved in their treatment decisions, although there is marked variation between individuals in how active a role they want to take, and in their need for detailed information (Table 18.5). It has been suggested that active involvement in decision-making may increase the effectiveness of treatment, and that all those involved in care should therefore facilitate this involvement by:

- Providing accurate information in clear and simple language that is relevant and meaningful to the individual, allowing time for them to assimilate it and ask questions.
- Determining how active the person wants to be in the decision-making Process.
- Assessing the person's knowledge of MS, and available treatments and services.
- Assessing complicating factors influencing decisions, which include cognitive impairment related to MS, and depression or anxiety (which may need treatment first).

In doing so there is a need to:

- Recognize the need for flexibility in approach, including the range of formats and levels of information that might need to be provided.
- Establish a practical working relationship with the person with MS.
- Acknowledge that the amount of involvement should reflect the person's needs and wishes.
- Acknowledge that different types and sources of information have variable effects on patient decisions.

CHAPTER 18 PRINCIPLES OF ONGOING MANAGEMENT **181**

Table 18.5 Patient preferences for involvement in decision making

Level of involvement	Description
Pure autonomy	The individual prefers to make the decision about which treatment they will receive
Informed choice	The individual prefers to make the decision about treatment after seriously considering the professional's opinion
Shared decision-making	The individual prefers to share responsibility with the professional for deciding which treatment is best
Professional as agent	The individual prefers the professional to make the final decision about treatment, but to seriously consider their opinion
Paternalistic	The individual prefers to leave all decisions regarding treatment to the professional

After Degner LF, Sloan JA, Venkatesh P. (1997) The Control Preferences Scale. *Canadian Journal of Nursing Research*; **29**: (3), 21–43.

Comprehensive assessment of needs

Assessment is central to effective management. A detailed, accurate and comprehensive assessment of the needs of the person with MS and their carer is essential to determine whether specific areas may benefit from intervention at a specific point in time. This assessment process is most effective when undertaken by professionals with specialist knowledge of MS. Such an assessment provides the basis for the formulation and implementation of individual care plans according both to need and to the patient's personal preferences. In undertaking any assessment it is essential that 'hidden' problems, such as fatigue, depression, cognitive impairment, impaired sexual function or reduced bladder control, is included, as these are often important contributors to difficulties experienced. A standardized review checklist, which is used each time a person with MS starts a new episode of care, may be useful to remind the clinician of potential problems that the person may face (Table 18.6). Given the life long nature of MS, formal reassessments should be undertaken at appropriate intervals. Use of a standardized procedure such as the review checklist can also be useful for preventing duplication between professionals, and for the purposes of future comparison. It is of particular benefit where regular rotation of staff through a service may mean that the person is reviewed each time by a different person.

Table 18.6 Review checklist

Initial question

It is best to start by asking an open-ended question such as:

'Since you were last seen or assessed has any activity you used to undertake been limited, stopped or affected?'

Activity domains

Then, especially if nothing has been identified, it is worth asking questions directly, choosing those appropriate to the situation based on your knowledge of the person with MS from the list below:

'Are you still able to undertake, as far as you wish:
• Vocational activities (work, education, other occupation)?
• Leisure activities?
• Family roles?
• Shopping and other community activities?
• Washing, dressing, using the toilet?
• Getting about (either by walking or in other ways) and getting in and out of your house?
• Controlling your environment (opening doors, switching things on and off, using the phone)?'

If restrictions are identified, the reasons for these should be identified as far as possible considering impairments (see below), and social and physical factors.

Common impairments

It is worth asking about specific impairments from the list below, again adapting to the situation and what you already know:

'Since you were last seen have you developed any problems with:
• Fatigue, endurance, being overtired?
• Speech and communication?
• Balance and falling?
• Chewing and swallowing food and drink?
• Unintended change in weight?
• Pain or painful abnormal sensations?
• Control over your bladder and bowels?
• Control over your movement?
• Vision and your eyes?
• Thinking, remembering?
• Your mood?
• Your sexual function or partnership relations?
• How you get on in social situations?'

Final question

Finally, it is always worth finishing off with a further open-ended question:

'Are there any other new problems that you think might be due to MS that concern you?'

A positive answer to any of the above questions should lead to more detailed assessment and management.

Reproduced with permission from: *The NICE Guidelines for the Management of MS in primary and secondary care, Clinical Guideline 8*, p. 60, 2003.

Chapter 19

The role of the MS specialist nurse

MS specialist nurses work in a holistic way and are often the fulcrum of the multi-disciplinary team in MS care. Their roles are diverse. They provide information, support, and advice about the condition from time of diagnosis and throughout the disease spectrum; monitor and improve standards of care through supervision and audit; provide professional leadership; and develop MS management through teaching, application of research-based practice, and support to colleagues in other disciplines.

MS specialist nurses use a social model of disability and the concept of empowerment to guide their practice. They adopt a holistic, collaborative, and coordinated approach, in an attempt to enable people with MS to achieve their maximal potential towards self management.

The complexity of disablement and multiple sites of neurological damage in MS mean that there is a clear need for interdisciplinary teamwork; joint care planning and 'trouble shooting' of patient problems as well as joint attendance at multidisciplinary clinics are commonplace in practice. The MS nurse has been described as a 'potential link-worker' in coordinating service provision for those living with MS.

A key role of the MS specialist nurse is to empower those affected by MS by providing a greater understanding of the condition. The role also involves acting as a consultant and educational resource for staff striving towards greater awareness and knowledge of MS in the health and social arena.

The essential skills of a specialist nurse practitioner are:
- Clinical leadership
- Research awareness
- Development of nursing knowledge
- Acting as consultant
- Educator
- Change agent
- Evaluating care.

These skills are detailed in Tables 19.1–5.

Table 19.1 As **clinical expert**, the MS specialist nurse must be able to:

- Deliver direct care to people with MS throughout the course of the disease from diagnosis to palliative care to death.
- Assess, plan, implement, review, and document individualized care plans.
- Lead nursing initiatives in the management of people with MS.
- Provide nursing assessment in the primary, secondary, and tertiary settings.
- Initiate and run nurse-led clinics.
- Acknowledge the expertise and experience of professional colleagues and the boundaries of their different roles.
- Provide telephone access offering advice, support and information to people with MS and their families, members of the multidisciplinary and primary care teams.
- Design care pathways appropriate to people with MS across the continuum of the disease.
- Identify areas for improvement and lead service developments.
- Create a service which is accessible and responsive to the needs of people with MS, and their families.
- Create a service that is appropriate for primary care groups, trusts, and members of the multidisciplinary team.

Table 19.2 As **consultant**, the MS specialist nurse must be able to:

- Liaise with primary care groups/trusts, offering advice, education, and support.
- Collaborate with medical staff in the assessment and management of symptoms, treatments, and complications of MS.
- Play a pivotal role within the multidisciplinary team, while recognizing boundaries of knowledge.
- Ensure the most appropriately skilled professional is consulted regarding the needs of individual patients.
- Foster a culture of trust and mutual support within the multidisciplinary team.
- Disseminate and share information, experience, and research findings with nurses and other members of the multidisciplinary team.
- Provide support and leadership to nursing colleagues and peer groups.
- Within the parameters of local employers' guidelines, promote awareness of MS and MS nursing by providing accurate information to the media.
- Liaise and work closely with MS charities and other relevant independent organisations.
- Contribute to planning MS services with primary care groups, local health care co-operatives, NHS hospital trusts, residential homes, and social services.

Table 19.3 As **educator**, the MS specialist nurse must be able to:

- Participate in educational programmes on MS for members of the multidisciplinary team, primary care groups, trusts, MS charities, professional organizations, and government bodies.
- Provide information, support and advice to healthcare team members and use adult learning principles to promote confidence in managing MS-related problems.
- Promote reflective practice by facilitating discussion about good practice and problem areas.
- Develop the knowledge base of health professionals, including generalist nurses, using models of empowerment.
- Promote the role of the nurse within the multidisciplinary team by role clarification through professional communication.
- Promote nursing skills of assessment and practice to medical colleagues by using good verbal communication skills and concise accurate documentation.
- Share information and learning with colleagues through presentations at local, national, and international conferences.
- Promote patient education by encouraging responsibility for health and well-being and emphasising the concept of 'wellness' using appropriate literature and communication methods.
- Ensure patient education strategies are based on health promotion models, not traditional medical models.
- Facilitate patient empowerment by promoting advocacy, facilitation and networking amongst people with MS.
- Encourage and facilitate the implementation of public health legislation, ensuring that this is reflected in local policy and practice.

Table 19.4 In **research**, the MS specialist nurse must be able to:

- Identify areas in nursing practice from which clear clinical questions can be formulated.
- Develop and share critical appraisal skills systematically to review and question the research process.
- Develop an understanding of the processes involved in evidence-based care, and a knowledge of where to obtain evidence.
- Identify the process necessary to implement and incorporate relevant findings into practice.
- Understand the barriers to using evidence-based care in the health care setting.
- Continue to measure performance against expected outcomes.
- Initiate and/or cooperate with colleagues in research into MS nursing.
- Disseminate nursing research findings to colleagues.

Table 19.5 Within a **clinical governance** framework, the MS specialist nurse has a key role in delivering high quality services within the following areas:

Monitoring

Quality standards as a result of a national inspectorate, the Commission for Health Improvement (CHI), the new National Performance Framework and national patient and user survey. MS specialist nurses must play an active part in the clinical governance process.

Clinical audit

The MS specialist nurse should participate in clinical audit programmes, which embrace a multidisciplinary approach and address important quality issues that will improve both the patients' experience and outcome.

Clinical effectiveness

MS specialist nurses need to develop their research appraisal skills and have access to information to ensure that their practice is based on the best available evidence. In addition, MS specialist nurses should endeavour to share examples of best practice with others as well as participating in clinical practice benchmarking as a means of achieving consistently high standards across organizational boundaries.

Clinical risk management

MS specialist nurses should have a clear understanding of local policies, which aim to minimize and manage the risks associated with adverse incidents. MS specialist nurses should have access to relevant clinical guidelines to support appropriate decision-making and ensure good outcomes for the patient.

Quality assurance

The MS specialist nurse is likely to be exposed to a range of quality activities, which attempt to monitor and measure performance. These will include standard setting and developing care pathways. An understanding of the local complaints procedure will provide further guidance.

Staff and organizational development

MS specialist nurses should participate in regular appraisal to identify and agree training and development needs, and their practice should be guided by professional self-regulation. They should encourage an organizational culture that fosters openness and an ability to learn from mistakes, rather than apportioning blame.

Chapter 20

Rehabilitation concepts and principles

Definitions of rehabilitation

There is often confusion about the meaning of the term rehabilitation, making it difficult at times to distinguish it from other forms of care and support. In part this is because rehabilitation is often a function of services, rather than necessarily being a service in its own right. This can be illustrated by the following range of definitions of rehabilitation, which highlight the ongoing and all-encompassing nature of rehabilitation. By necessity therefore it is crucial that rehabilitation is viewed as a concept (as distinct from a service) which should underpin all services dealing with people with MS throughout the lifelong course of the disease.

The following examples provide a flavour of the different definitions which are available to describe rehabilitation:

'Rehabilitation is an active process of change by which a person who has become disabled acquires and uses the knowledge and skill necessary for optimal physical, psychological and social function'[1].

'Rehabilitation means a goal directed and time-limited process aimed at enabling an impaired person to reach optimum mental, physical and social functioning, thus providing him with the tools to change his own life.'[2]

'Rehabilitation is a problem solving process by which those who are disabled by injury or disease achieve a full recovery or if a full recovery is not possible realize their optimal physical, mental and social potential and are integrated into their most appropriate environment.'[3]

Intrinsic to all of these definitions, and to the philosophy of rehabilitation is that:

- The primary focus is on the behavioural aspects of illness, where the key objective is on the restoration of the maximum degree possible either of function (physical or mental), or role (within the family, social network or workforce).
- To be effective, rehabilitation needs to be responsive to users' needs and wishes by ensuring that the affected person and their family become central to planning and actively participating in it.
- It has a strong educational bias which aims to equip the person with effective coping skills so that they can manage deficits and apply solutions to challenges.
- It usually requires a mixture of clinical, social, therapeutic interventions that also address issues relevant to a person's physical and social environment.
- It is characterized by coordinated and coherent teamworking between different professionals who work within a coherent model of illness, and who are aware of each other's roles and the ways that interventions may interact with others.

Rehabilitation should be viewed as a constantly evolving and ongoing process which is relevant and applicable at every stage of the condition from initial diagnosis to the management of severe disability. It is not

1 Disability Committee of the Royal College of Physicians (1981). London, HMSO.
2 United Nations World Programme of Action Concerning Disabled persons, 1983.
3 World Health Organization (1980). *International Classification of Impairments, Disabilities and Handicaps.* Geneva, WHO.

uncommon for health professionals to believe that in the more advanced stages of the disease people with moderate or severe disability are unable to benefit from interventions aimed at improving their level of function and mobility. There is evidence from a range of clinical trials to demonstrate that this is not the case. It is the responsibility of health professionals to be aware of both the specific and broader aspects of management, such as rehabilitation interventions, which may improve the quality of life of all those affected by the disease.

Multi-disciplinary team approach

Effective teamwork occurs when a group of people work together as an integrated whole to achieve a truly holistic approach to management. It occurs when the work of each person is supported by, and in turn supports and reinforces, the work of others. The important features of an effective team have been well documented in the literature and are listed in Table 20.1.

Despite the fact that these features are relatively easily identifiable, and that there is widespread agreement that a team approach is key to successful ongoing management, the reality in practice is that teamworking frequently fails to occur. It often seems difficult for those involved to put their own personal and political agendas to one side in order to work collaboratively either within or across organizational boundaries, to provide care based on the individual needs of the patient. Perhaps this is not surprising given the large number and wide variety of different disciplines who may be involved in the care of people with MS (Table 20.2)

It is increasingly recognized that effective management of people with long-term conditions requires a collaborative team work approach across the broad continuum of care. This approach aims to ensure that the right professional is involved at the right time and in the right place, with the patient and family acting as consultants to the team. This clearly further broadens the concept of what has traditionally been viewed as the multidisciplinary team, as it involves collaborative working by people from both health and social service organizations as well as other statutory organisations. This provides enormous challenges for all those involved in care.

There are a number of practical strategies which can help to facilitate teamwork. These include:
- Joint goal setting
- Regular team meetings
- Case conferences
- Key workers
- Joint documentation (this may be in the form of patient held records, particularly in the community setting; or integrated care pathways)
- The use of a common conceptual framework and vocabulary to enhance communication (for instance the World Health Organization's International Classification of Functioning, Disability and Health
- Integrated care pathways
- Shared geographical spaces, such as shared offices
- Opportunities for mutual support and enjoyment, which include social occasions outside of the work arena.

These are most easily implemented when the team involved is sited within a single organization.

Table 20.1 Characteristics of an effective team

- Shared goals
- Mutual respect and equality for team members
- Effective communication
- Transparent decision making
- Effective leadership
- Interdependence
- Cooperation and collaboration
- Coordination of activities
- Division of effort
- Avoids duplication of effort
- Allows each discipline to contribute its own knowledge and skill to patient goals
- Role clarification
- Shared responsibilities
- Team unity.

Table 20.2 Disciplines and services typically involved in MS care

Disciplines	Services
• General practitioners • Neurologists • Nurses (including specialist MS nurses) • Occupational therapists • Orthoptists • Podiatrists • Physiotherapists (including specialist MS therapists) • Clinical psychologists • Social workers • Speech and language therapists	• Continence advisory and management services • Dietetics services • Ophthamology services • Orthotics services • Pain management services • Specialist wheelchair and seating services

The International Classification of Functioning, Disability and Health

In order to have a coherent and comprehensive approach to rehabilitation management it is necessary for people from different disciplines, who may be working in different services and different organisations to communicate effectively with one another. For this to occur they need to share a common conceptual framework and vocabulary. The World Health Organization's International Classification of Functioning Disability and Health (ICF) provides a very useful conceptual framework for describing, planning and evaluating MS services. It enables a standardized language to be used when talking about the problems that people face as a consequence of their disease. This model, with definition of key terms, is shown in Table 20.3.

In essence the ICF model allows the description of a person's health situation at 4 different levels:

• The disease
• The signs and symptoms
• The person's behaviour
• The person's social situation.

It recognizes 3 different contextual factors:

• Social environment
• Physical environment
• The person's internal environment (beliefs and expectations).

In doing so, it enables a comprehensive assessment to be undertaken. This can enhance clinicians' potential to address these issues in a systematic and logical manner.

Table 20.3 The World Health Organization's International Classification of Functioning, Disability and Health

Level of illness

Term	Synonym	Definition
Pathology	Disease/diagnosis	Abnormalities in the structure and/or function of an organ or organ system.
Impairment	Symptoms/signs	Abnormalities of psychological, physiological, or anatomical structure and/or function. These are the presenting signs and symptoms such as fatigue, spasticity, weakness, depression, or memory loss.
Activity (previously disability)	Function/observed behaviour	Abnormalities, changes or restrictions in function, such as in dressing, washing, feeding, and general mobility.
Participation (previously handicap)	Social position/roles	Abnormalities, changes or restrictions in involvement in life situations. Difficulties may result in the person fulfilling their role, for instance as a parent, or participating in their preferred work and leisure interests.

Contextual factors

Domain	Examples	
Personal	Previous illness of self or others	This mainly refers to attitudes, beliefs and expectations. These often arise from past experience of illness, but also relate to personal characteristics such as personal outlook and reasoning style.
Physical	House, local shops, carers	This mainly refers to local physical structures but also to resources such as carers.
Social	Friends, family, laws	This mainly refers to legal and local cultural issues, including the expectation of others.

Adapted from Wade DT, Green Q (2001). *A study of services of multiple sclerosis; lessons for managing chronic disability* 2001. London, Royal College of Physicians.

Goal setting

Key to successful management is the notion that people are actively engaged in managing their condition because they see the process as being directly relevant and meaningful to them. Goal setting is a practical means of facilitating this involvement. Furthermore, it provides a structured and objective way of planning and monitoring progress, both for staff and those affected by MS. In doing so it can help to ensure that management remains focused and patient centred.

Goal setting involves skill, time and effort. In brief, there are a number of fundamental principles to successful goal setting:

- There should be active involvement of the person with MS and their family so that the goals are relevant and motivating.
- The goals should be understandable and accessible to the person— this requires the language used to be unambiguous and jargon-free.
- Goals should be SMART (refer to Table 20.4)
- Goals should cover both short-term and long-term outcomes. There should be a logical stepwise progression in the development of goals, with short-term goals leading to the achievement of long-term goals.
- Goals should express what is wanted to be accomplished in behavioural terms. For example, rather than a goal 'to strengthen lower limb muscles', it should be focused on a behaviour such as 'being able to climb one flight of stairs independently within x days'.
- Goals should be written in positive terms, for example 'to reduce dependency in dressing' is better expressed as 'being able to fasten buttons without help within X weeks'.
- Before setting goals all those involved should have an awareness of the factors that impact on goal achievement. These factors include: cognitive function, mood, and environmental factors such as availability of resources. This can help focus the goals and make achievement more likely.
- Studies show that regular and specific feedback to the person about goal achievement (or failure) is essential to improve performance.
- If a goal is not achieved, the reasons for non achievement should be identified.

When writing goals there are some key elements to consider:

- Long-term goals should state the expected level of function in broad terms.
- In contrast short-term goals describe the immediate steps to achieving long-term goals. They should clearly describe:
  - *Who* will perform the behaviour; typically this is the person, but sometimes is the carer.
  - *What* the person will do (the activity).
  - *Under what conditions* (the environmental conditions).
  - *How well* they will do it (for example level of assistance, number of attempts, aids used); and
  - *By when* the activity will have been completed (the time scale for achievement).

Table 20.4 Characteristics of SMART goals

SMART goals are those which are:

Specific—they should not be broad based or vague.

Measurable—they should be written so that there is no doubt as to whether they have been met (i.e. they can allow a yes or no answer when evaluated).

Achievable—they should be challenging but achievable.

Relevant—agreed as relevant and important by the person with MS.

Time limited—a specific time period for achievement should be stated.

Goal setting can at times be very complex. It is important to acknowledge that disagreements can arise during the goal setting process. Patients, families and professionals, while sharing some concerns, also have different perspectives. For example:

• People with MS themselves usually want to make their own decisions. They know their own lifestyle best, habits and support systems, and the amount of energy they wish to expend on aspects of health care such as therapy and retraining. At times this may conflict with the views of professionals and carers.

• Sometimes family members feel that they are more objective than the person with MS in assessing their needs. It should be recognized however that they may also have distorted views re: the person's capabilities and desires.

• Professionals generally want to provide 'excellent' treatment. They may find it difficult to permit patients and families to do things their own way, especially if they feel that time, money and effort are wasted, or needlessly poor outcome may result. As a consequence clinicians may be tempted to usurp decision-making power in the enthusiasm for providing optimal care.

An awareness of these issues will help clinicians to find out what peoples' real goals are and help them to achieve them. They are a useful means of making the expectations of people transparent from the beginning of the rehabilitation process, rather than at the end! Decisions about the goals of intervention sometimes requires negotiation, and compromises may need to be made by any of those involved in the process.

Chapter 21

Approaches to rehabilitation

The provision of rehabilitation for people with MS can broadly be described as falling into three main categories:
- Education and health promotion
- Restorative rehabilitation
- Maintenance rehabilitation.

When viewed together they can be seen as providing a continuum of rehabilitation care in which a different emphasis is placed on different aspects of the rehabilitation process throughout different stages of the disease.

Health promotion

Health promotion is as important to people with MS as it is to the general population. It is therefore essential that it is incorporated as a routine part of healthcare delivery. This involves:
- Encouraging people to maintain a positive attitude that is wellness oriented rather than disease oriented.
- Facilitating people to participate in the wide range of health promoting activities that the general population participate in, and which include maintaining a healthy diet and controlling weight.
- Providing advice and opportunities for people to participate in exercise programmes. It is now widely acknowledged that regular moderate exercise in people with MS is important to reduce the risk of coronary disease, lower blood pressure, help to protect against osteoporosis, and to play a role in reducing stress and low mood. Schemes such as the general practitioner referred 'Exercise on prescription schemes'[1] are one mechanism for facilitating this. In these schemes people are referred by their GP for supervised exercise programmes, often within the community at facilities such as local leisure centres or gyms.
- Ensuring that people pay attention to the broad array of health measures that are undertaken in the general population, such as blood pressure measurement, breast examination, cervical screening, prostate examination, blood sugar level, cholesterol and lipids.
- Provide ongoing support so that they can access accurate advice and helpful information to help them self-manage the wide array of symptoms they may face.

---

1 Department of Health (2001). *Exercise referral systems: A national quality assurance framework.* Available at: http://www.dh.gov.uk/PublicationsAndStatistics/Publications

Restorative rehabilitation

In general people are referred for formal rehabilitation after they have lost an important function, or are experiencing difficulty maintaining their usual roles, either due to acute changes following a relapse, or to deterioration as a consequence of disease progression. Restorative rehabilitation focuses on maximizing quality of life by restoring lost abilities so as to enable the person to function at their optimal capacity within the limits of their disease.

Typically this type of rehabilitation is provided when the level of disability is mild to moderate. The rehabilitation episode is time limited, relatively short in duration, and is aimed at achieving specific measurable goals, with success often being measured in fairly concrete terms of improvements in functional ability. It can be provided within an inpatient setting (either acute hospital or a rehabilitation unit), as an outpatient, or within the community.

Improvements can be achieved through a variety of different interventions which include those aimed at:

- Directly improving existing physical, emotional and cognitive impairments, such as improving strength and range of motion; reducing hypertonicity, reducing depression, and improving bladder and bowel control.
- Involving processes that include learning, the acquisition of new skills and the changing of behaviour. These strategies tend to be used when impairments cannot be reversed.

As highlighted in Chapter 18 (Principles of ongoing management), unlike in acute and reversible illnesses, rehabilitation in MS is never a 'one off'. A key aim of rehabilitation in MS is to help the person adjust to and cope with the varying disabling consequences of the disease, by adapting and readapting to MS repeatedly over time. It is therefore often appropriate that, during the course of the disease, restorative rehabilitation is undertaken on a repeated basis, by different services, and across a variety of different settings. The key factor for determining whether and when further restorative rehabilitation is required is that clearly identifiable goals can be set that can be achieved over a time limited period.

Maintenance rehabilitation

Maintenance rehabilitation aims to maintain function within the limits of the progression of the disease by optimizing health. This requires, wherever possible, preventing avoidable and unwanted secondary complications from developing, or arresting and improving them if they occur. This is important since both reduced function and secondary complications (which include contractures, pressure sores, depression, disuse weakness, unemployment, and carer ill-health) are costly both in economic and quality of life terms.

As is characteristic of any rehabilitation approach, a multidisciplinary team is involved in providing a wide range of interventions, which can be focused at different levels including:

- Impairments, by focusing on aspects such as the implementation of regimens to maintain or improve cardiovascular fitness, range of motion, strength, pressure care, and postural alignment; or by providing counselling and emotional support where necessary.
- Function, for example by maintaining independence through the education of optimal movement patterns, the use of aids and equipment, or by ensuring adequate personal help is provided.
- Preservation of safety, for example in functions such as transfers.

Too often people with MS are referred for maintenance rehabilitation in the later stages of the disease, when disability is severe and when secondary complications have already become well established. This can mean that management is extremely difficult, very time consuming, and success is often limited. A further challenge to effective management is that maintenance rehabilitation is commonly provided within the community, either in the patient's own home or in long term institutional care. In these environments organisation of care and communication between staff is often complicated by the fact that the team members involved are usually large in number and include qualified and unqualified staff from both healthcare and social service organisations. Ensuring that input from such a diverse range of people across different organisations occurs appropriately and to a high standard is fraught with difficulties and raises numerous challenges, which include; determining how best to organize ongoing training; ensuring clear communication with regard to changes in circumstances and routines; and establishing common protocols for care. The case management approach is one way of attempting to tackle these difficulties, particularly in people with more complex and long term needs.

Although considered a high priority by people with MS and their carers, funding for the provision of services designed to deliver maintenance rehabilitation over the longer term is difficult to attain. This is not helped by the fact that little evidence exists to demonstrate its benefit. As a consequence the burden of long term care and maintenance therapy often falls on the carer, and carer burnout and emotional distress is common. Sustained follow-up services should be provided in order to prevent this situation from arising by monitoring patients health status, identifying potential complications and checking and reinforcing the implementation of care plans (Chapter 22).

Models of care and organization of service delivery

Introduction

The lifelong nature of MS, its variable course, the multiplicity and diversity of problems that may exist, and the subsequent wide variety of care needs, demands broad based, dynamic and collaborative models of care involving many professionals in health and allied services. It requires a comprehensive and flexible model of care, which enables different pathways of care to be available through a diverse range of services. These services may include:

- General practitioner services
- Inpatient and outpatient hospital services
- Rehabilitation units
- Community based services, including health and social services
- Links to a regional specialist neuroscience centre
- Links to voluntary and charitable organizations.

No single one of these settings or services can adequately meet a person's needs across the lifelong course of MS. Instead individuals need to access different services, for different reasons, at different points in time. An inevitable consequence of this is that people need to be transferred between services and organisations. This often results in fragmentation of the delivery of care, and it is not uncommon for confusion and anxiety to arise in patients, carers and professionals alike.

While these problems are common to the management of all neurological disorders, they are often magnified in MS due to the unpredictability and variability of the condition. Managing this complexity in practice is extremely difficult, and unfortunately there are no easy solutions to these problems since it requires a multiplicity of agencies, professions and services to work together, even though they are all funded, managed and held accountable though different means. A coherent 'whole systems' approach to the delivery of care attempts to address the fragmentation of care delivery by advocating that all parts of the healthcare system, social services and other statutory services have joint responsibility for care, and should work collaboratively using agreed protocols, to ensure that all of the services are working towards achieving a common 'patient centred' goal. Table 26.1 provides a schema of this system of care delivery.

Table 22.1 Services for people with MS: A collaborative 'whole systems' approach to care delivery

Hospital	Intensive rehabilitation	Intermediate services	Community based services
Diagnostic clinics	Specialist inpatient rehabilitation units	Community hospitals	General practice
Outpatient clinics, e.g.: • Assessment clinics • Relapse clinics • Spasticity clinics • Continence services	General inpatient rehabilitation units	Respite care services	Community rehabilitation within the person's home setting
Inpatient hospital stay, e.g. for relapse management; surgical procedures such as intrathecal baclofen pumps			Links with specialist vocational services; assessments within the work-place; liaison with local employment services
Outpatient therapy input, e.g. • Physiotherapy • Occupational therapy			Links with social services providing personal care and support within the person's home
			Links with voluntary organizations, e.g. MS Society
			Day hospitals
			Links with local leisure centres

Reproduced with permission from Freeman JA (2006). Service delivery and models of care in multiple sclerosis. In *Neurological Rehabilitation of Multiple Sclerosis* p. 145. Queen Square Neurological Rehabilitation Series (2006), Infoma UK Ltd.

Care pathways

No two people with MS are the same. The goal of care pathways is to make sure that the individual with MS receives the best care, in the best place, from the best person or team, at the best time.

Clinical need is clearly a key consideration when making decisions about where care should be best delivered for the person with MS. It is however not the only factor to consider. The physical, cognitive and emotional needs of the individual and their family/carers should also be taken into account. For instance the personal preferences of the person with MS, and lifestyle issues such as family and work considerations are key to the decision making process, but often appear to be neglected in practice. Staff must also consider the psychological impact of aspects such as the health care setting and the timing of interventions (such as rehabilitation) upon the person and how this might affect their ability or desire to actively participate in the process. Economic and practical considerations will also play a role in determining the chosen care pathway. For instance the team needs to consider physical factors within the treatment settings that will affect the intervention, such as the staff resources available both in terms of skill level and staff numbers, how much time is available for assessment and management, or how much assistance can be accessed for more complex situations. All of these are important considerations in determining the optimum pathway of care for an individual.

Often a number of options exist with regard to the pathway of care available to a person:

- During an acute attack, for example, steroid therapy in collaboration with rehabilitation could be provided either within a hospital environment or within the person's own home.
- Where the problems are complex and interrelated, a period of inpatient rehabilitation may be the optimal choice of management, enabling intensive daily multidisciplinary input to achieve improvements.
- On some occasions an inpatient admission might be far from ideal and perhaps even counterproductive. For instance, when the main aim of intervention is to teach the carer a suitable technique to help care for their severely disabled spouse, rehabilitation within the home environment is likely to be more relevant and effective.
- In other instances when the problems experienced are relatively straightforward, outpatient intervention may be effective in addressing problems while having the advantage of enabling home and work life to continue relatively undisturbed.

For many people, access to all of these services may be necessary at some stage of the disease course. Determining which service and approach best meets the needs of the individual at a specific point in time, requires a comprehensive assessment of needs from someone who has specialist experience and skill as well as local knowledge about the various options that are available. It requires those involved to reflect upon and answer a number of rather simple but searching questions (Table 22.2).

Table 22.2 Questions to consider when determining which pathway of care is most appropriate for an individual

- What care is required to meet this person's needs?
- Who is the most appropriate person/service to provide the care?
- When is the best time to give the care?
- What is the ideal place to deliver the care?
- How long is care likely to be needed?
- What systems are in place to check that this person's needs have been met, both in the short and longer term?

Methods of review

Given the lifelong nature of MS, and the fact that new symptoms can arise quite suddenly and unexpectedly, it is important that systems are in place which enable the patient's health status to be monitored, potential complications to be identified, and progress to be checked and reinforced on implementation of the care plan. This requires that services can respond in a timely and flexible way to people's needs. There are a variety of different methods in use for providing ongoing support, some of which include:

- Pre-scheduled outpatient clinic appointments
- Self-referral or open access systems
- Self-referral systems supplemented by scheduled return visits
- Telephone contact.

Pre-scheduled outpatient clinic appointments

It is common practice for people to be reviewed by their neurologist and other relevant health professionals at a pre-set interval, typically of 6 to 12 months, regardless of current need. While this can be helpful in managing symptoms which are insidiously progressive, it is of limited benefit either in proactively managing symptoms, or in responding to those with more intermittent, acute or complex needs. Furthermore there are often tight time constraints with outpatient appointments, which mean that there is little time to spend with an individual, or to involve relevant members of the multidisciplinary team. Finally, although one-stop-shops do exist, where a multidisciplinary service is provided on one site, this is relatively uncommon. More often it is the case that each professional schedules an independent review appointment. As a consequence it can be the case that the patient attends three or four separate 'annual reviews' by different professionals in consecutive months! It is perhaps not surprising therefore, that as a consequence of some or all of these issues, dissatisfaction with pre-scheduled outpatient clinics is expressed by users of the service.

Self-referral or open access systems

Self-referral or open access systems allow individuals the flexibility to access services when their needs change. In order for this system to be effective, people with MS and their carers need to know how, why and when they should contact services, should new problems arise. In essence, self-referral allows people to self-manage, but ensures they know whom to contact if advice or intervention is needed. With an increasing recognition that routine appointments can be a waste of time and resources, as well as failing to meet people's needs, the self-referral method of review is now being used to a greater extent, particularly within nursing and therapy services. This access does not always need to be in the form of a face-to-face appointment. Telephone helplines are now being used by some services to enable people with MS to access advice, usually from a specialist MS nurse. Some services have implemented the use of mobile telephones so that patients can receive a quick response when they need it.

The adoption of a rehabilitation approach, wherein people affected by MS are educated about the disease process, and about why and how things go astray, clearly goes some way to ensure that people will access services appropriately. Written information leaflets, which provide a flowchart of the decision making process for contacting specific services, can also be helpful in clarifying this and providing a memory prompt. Figure 22.1 provides an example of a flowchart, which can be embedded within a patient information leaflet, to help describe the decision making process for self-referral to a service such as physiotherapy.

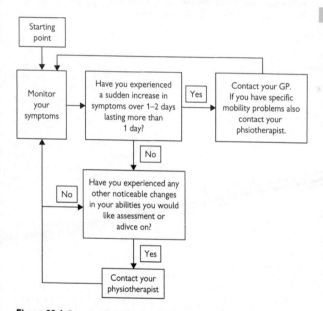

Figure 22.1 Example of a flowchart for monitoring symptoms and identifying who to contact.

Reproduced with permission from South Devon Health Services Physiotherapy Department.

Self-referral supplemented by scheduled return visits

While self-referral systems may suit many people, there are some who will not be able to engage appropriately in the self-referral decision making process, nor have confidence in it. Such people may include those with cognitive problems, depression, or those who lack self confidence in their own decision making abilities. It may also be less suitable for those with more complex physical issues such as severe spasticity and/or spasms which heighten the risk of the development of secondary complications such as pressure sores or contractures. The incorporation of regular planned face-to-face reviews may be an important safety net for these individuals. Increasingly, telephone reviews are also being used to supplement scheduled return visits or open access systems.

Chapter 23

Specialist regional neurological services

Introduction

It is now generally accepted that complex conditions, such as MS, are best managed by a combination of regional specialist and local services. Regional specialist services appear to be particularly beneficial when needs are complex, and where it is important that health professionals are seeing enough patients to understand the difficult issues encountered, and to develop and maintain the necessary skill level. It is also argued that specialised services reorganize care in a more efficient and effective manner, by bringing together the personnel and resources required to meet the patient's needs. Importantly there is some evidence to suggest that patients are also more satisfied and confident with the care they receive from specialist services.

These specialist regional services include:

- Specialist outpatient services based around the management of complex issues such as diagnosis and relapse management.
- Specialist outpatient services based around the management of complex symptoms such as spasticity and continence.
- Specialist outpatient services based around complex interventions such as wheelchair and seating, orthotics and functional electrical stimulation.
- Specialist units who provide an information, advice and assessment service for driving.
- Specialist inpatient neurological rehabilitation units.
- Specialist community rehabilitation teams.

National Guidelines for MS recommend that any person with MS whose symptoms or disability is persistent or troublesome, and not quickly and easily resolved, should be seen by an appropriate specialist service, such as some of those described above. Multiple referrals to these specialist services can, at times, be necessary over the course of the disease.

Referral mechanisms differ within different Trusts, and hence local policies are necessary so that all concerned know who is responsible for different aspects of care, and how it can be accessed. Local directories which provide contact and referral information about services relevant to MS have been developed in some areas. These directories go some way to helping all those involved in care to negotiate the complicated network of health and social service systems which exist. They can help to facilitate patients in becoming more proactive in their management by enabling them, for instance, to have informed discussions with clinicians such as general practitioners about the services available which they may wish to access.

A brief description of some of the key specialist neurological services follows, together with some examples of successful models of practice.

Demyelinating disease diagnostic clinics

Diagnostic clinics are designed to facilitate accurate and timely diagnosis of MS through expert clinical assessment and access to key diagnostic tests. Research findings suggest that, in addition to receiving an accurate diagnosis, people with MS need support, information, education and guidance in order to adapt effectively to the impact of the disease. The neurologist and the MS nurse specialist are key in providing this at this early stage. It appears that the quality of care received at the time of diagnosis significantly influences the ability of the person with MS to begin to successfully adapt to the impact of the disease, and to begin to develop a lifelong collaborative working relationship with healthcare professionals. Many believe that the foundations of this relationship should be cemented at the diagnostic stage. Table 23.1 provides an example of a model of good practice for a demyelinating diagnostic clinic.

Table 23.1 Case study 1

Demyelinating Disease Diagnostic Clinic, National Hospital for Neurology and Neurosurgery, London, UK

The Demyelinating Disease Diagnostic Clinic (DDC) investigates people suspected of having a demyelinating disease, primarily MS. The clinic was modelled on the UK Multiple Sclerosis Society diagnostic phase standards. GPs and neurologists refer people suspected of having MS to the clinic.

The DDC aims to minimize the time between referral and completion of tests by offering same day tests and follow-up within 4 weeks. The clinic allocates a 45 minute initial appointment with the consultant neurologist and MS nurse and provides access to key diagnostic tests for MS, as appropriate. Follow-up appointments for all people are scheduled to allow 45 minutes with the neurologist and MS nurse followed by a further 30 minutes with the MS nurse in a quiet room.

The DDC provides continuity so that people see the same doctor and nurse, and provides access to professionals with expertise in MS. The structure provides an appropriate setting and experienced professional support to deal with the initial psychological impact of the diagnosis. The clinic offers ongoing support through health promotion and self-management programmes.

All newly diagnosed people and their families are offered one-to-one appointments, and have access to a structured educational programme 'Working together to understand multiple sclerosis'.

An audit of the service showed shorter waiting times from referral to first appointment and faster receipt of investigation results, when compared with two existing diagnostic service models within the same hospital (the general neurology clinic and the inpatient investigation unit).[1]

Source: http://www.dh.gov.uk/PolicyAndGuidance/HealthAndSocialCareTopics/LongTermConditions/BestPractice Accessed April 2006.

1 Porter B, Thompson A (2001). Management of the diagnostic phase of multiple sclerosis: a comparison of three models. *Multiple Sclerosis* **7**: S120.

MS relapse clinics

Planned, coordinated multidisciplinary team assessment and management of relapses through the use of MS relapse clinics has been shown to improve outcome. The aim of these clinics is to provide rapid access to any patient experiencing a relapse, and to provide them with a full multidisciplinary team assessment at one visit, followed by a decision on optimal relapse management. Table 23.2 provides an example of a model of good practice for an MS relapse clinic.

Table 23.2 Case study 2

The Walton Centre for Neurology and Neurosurgery, Liverpool, UK

This clinic was established after research conducted by Craig et al.[1] demonstrated that patients in relapse who were treated with steroids combined with planned multidisciplinary team management fared better than a control group who received standard neurology or day ward management of their relapse. These benefits were in terms of motor impairment, disability and handicap.

The service provides:

- rapid access to an assessment clinic within the existing MS clinic, through the specific allocation of four appointment slots each week for people who are in relapse.
- a co-ordinated, multidisciplinary approach and improved planning for rehabilitation when steroid treatment is advocated medically. The team comprises a physiotherapist, occupational therapist, MS specialist nurse, an orthoptist, a registrar and a consultant neurologist.
- the development of a treatment plan agreed between the patient and the multi-disciplinary team.
- close links with outside agencies to ensure appropriate monitoring and follow-up of patients during steroid treatment.

The service uses a number of outcome measures and feedback forms to undertake service evaluation.

Source: http://www.dh.gov.uk/PolicyAndGuidance/HealthAndSocialCareTopics/LongTermConditions/ BestPractice Accessed April 2006.

1 Craig J et al (2003). A randomized controlled trial comparing rehabilitation against standard therapy in multiple sclerosis patients receiving intravenous steroid treatment. Journal of Neurology Neurosurgery and Psychiatry; **74**: 1255–30.

Spasticity services

Spasticity services consolidate and centralize treatment for people with spasticity by bringing together a team of professionals skilled in assessing and treating spasticity into one clinic. Without them the person with spasticity frequently has to access a number of different services in an attempt to deal with their problems. Typically the person undergoes a comprehensive assessment by a core team, who usually include a neurologist, physiotherapist and specialist nurse. This is followed by discussion of the findings with the patient, the development of goals and formulation of recommendations. The team and patient then arrive at a treatment plan, which may include medications, therapies, injections, or a combination of these. The establishment of these specialist services provides the opportunity for the relevant members of the team to discuss difficult to manage, and often long term problems in detail. These discussions between specialties are usually invaluable in decision making. Table 23.3 provides an example of a model of good practice for a spasticity service.

Table 23.3 Case study 3

The Spasticity Service, The National Hospital for Neurology and Neurosurgery, London

This service offers comprehensive multidisciplinary assessment, treatment and follow-up to patients with spasticity at all stages of the pathway from diagnosis and education through to palliative care. The core team consists of a consultant neurologist, a clinical specialist physiotherapist and 2 clinical nurse specialists, with input from a neurophysiologist and anaesthetist.

Once a referral is received, an integrated care pathway (ICP) is begun so that by the time the patient is seen in the assessment clinic, information will have been collected from all health and social care professionals involved with the patient's care, and follow-up outpatient physiotherapy arranged if appropriate, e.g. for patients suitable for botulinum toxin therapy. Use of the ICP ensures that, for most patients, a single clinic visit is sufficient for assessment and initial management.

A variety of treatments for spasticity are available including botulinum toxin, functional electrical stimulation, and intrathecal therapies. The team has developed a number of protocols and treatment algorithms which they are willing to share.

The team is involved in research, and are members of the European group 'SPASM', which aims to establish best practice in the measurement of spasticity based on current knowledge and research.

Source:
http://www.dh.gov.uk/PolicyAndGuidance/HealthAndSocialCareTopics/LongTermConditions/BestPractice/CommunityRehabilitation Accessed April 2006.

Continence advisory services

The National Clinical Guidelines on MS management (2003) recommend that any person with MS who, despite treatment, has incontinence more than once a week should be referred to a specialist continence service. These services provide a 'one stop' clinic for the assessment, treatment and management of bladder and bowel problems problems, and as a source for links to other services. They enable people with continence problems to access the service of any of the disciplines within the team through one initial referral. Typically these disciplines include the neurologist, urologist, and continence nurse. The continence assessment is essential to establish the degree and type of continence problem. Following this a management plan and recommendations are made. This may be in the form of drug intervention, introduction of intermittent self-catheterization, or referral to the urologist for further investigations. Close liaison with the GP is seen as key to effectively planning a person's care.

Specialist wheelchair and seating services

The purpose of specialist wheelchair and seating services is to provide a centralized and 'one stop' service which can evaluate the individual needs of the person with complex disability in relation to posture and seating; and to recommend special seating equipment and adaptations to the wheelchair, which are necessary due to functional, postural, and/or skin considerations (Chapter 29, wheelchair and seating section, discusses this in more detail). Typically these regional services are comprised of teams of physiotherapists, occupational therapists, rehabilitation engineers, and technicians with expertise in this area of management and specialist knowledge in the wide range of equipment available. Specialist centres provide more complex equipment while simpler seating systems are prescribed by local wheelchair systems. Studies in other neurological conditions such as spinal cord injury have demonstrated that patients who attend specialist seating assessment clinics have better skin management, supporting the use of these clinics as a proactive intervention to improve patient independence, knowledge and awareness, and potentially reduce pressure ulcer incidence.

Functional electrical stimulation clinics

Specialist clinics for functional electrical stimulation (FES) are increasingly being developed. These clinics tend to be held within physiotherapy departments, rehabilitation units or orthotics services by staff who have received specific training on the application and use of these devices. In the vast majority of cases these clinics are not MS specific clinics, but deal with a variety of patients who have dropped foot as a result of upper motor neuron deficit. At the FES clinic people are assessed, and then providing they meet specific criteria (refer to assessment and treatment protocol available on *http://www.salisburyfes.com*), they are trialled with the FES device. In most cases an improvement in gait is immediately apparent. If this is the case, then the device is fitted, the user is taught how to apply and use the device and the stimulation is gradually increased over a period of a few weeks with input from health professionals as necessary to ensure safe and effective management. Follow-up is provided by the clinic at regular intervals.

Specialist driving assessment centres

Specialist regional driving assessment centres provide information, assessment and advice on driving for disabled and older people, their families and professionals. They undertake assessments to determine the person's safety to drive. They provide information and advice about a wide range of issues related to driving, including: the most suitable type of car to drive; any aids or adaptations that are required; sources of finance, purchase or hire of a vehicle; information about insurance for driving; and advice on alternative means of transport if driving is not possible. Many also provide a service for driving tuition, and many undertake the fitting of car adaptations.

Specialist regional inpatient neurological rehabilitation units

A specialist neuro-rehabilitation approach to the rehabilitation management of people with MS is strongly supported by current National Guidelines in the UK as well as by a range of internationally agreed expert consensus documents on rehabilitation in MS. In contrast to more common neurological conditions such as stroke, where disease specific rehabilitation units are seen as the gold standard, the incidence and prevalence of MS means that many health services lack the necessary critical mass of patients to justify the development of a condition specific service. As a consequence specialist neuro-rehabilitation units (as distinct from MS specific rehabilitation units) are recommended. In reality, practical factors such as the availability of specialist staff and facilities, means that there is usually a mixed approach to the provision of rehabilitation. The bulk of rehabilitation is delivered by generic rehabilitation or general neurological services (across hospital, inpatient rehabilitation and community settings), and is complemented by regional specialist neuro-rehabilitation services which specialise in neurologically based disability.

Referral for inpatient multidisciplinary rehabilitation is often chosen when the problems experienced are complex and interrelated, and where intensive daily multidisciplinary input is required over a period of time, to achieve improvements. One of the key advantages of an inpatient rehabilitation unit is that it provides the person with an opportunity to focus on their own rehabilitation needs, free from dealing with the everyday issues within their home life. It enables them to practice the skills or approaches learnt, and to receive detailed feedback on them, over the 24-hour period, with immediate access to rehabilitation staff for advice and assistance.

Differences in referral procedures and admission criteria exist between different units:

- Some services admit according to preset admission criteria, which may include the need for input from two or more disciplines, the need to be medically stable and the ability to participate in intensive therapy sessions.
- Some services undertake a multidisciplinary team assessment to identify who may benefit from inpatient admission—integral to this process is the identification of areas of potential improvement and the establishment of achievable goals, agreed by both the patient and the team, prior to admission.
- Other units admit on the basis of the referrer's assessment for the need for rehabilitation input. Typically the referrer is either the neurologist or the general practitioner.

Currently there is no robust evidence to support one approach over another.

Table 23.4 Typical rehabilitation interventions

- Treatment of any reversible underlying impairment, such as weakness, loss of range, altered tone.
- Task-related practice of specific activities.
- Provision of suitable equipment, with training in its use.
- Altering the environment as needed, and making recommendations re: potential alterations within the home environment.
- Teaching others how to assist with, or take over, tasks.
- Providing education and advice about how to prevent difficulties from arising wherever possible, or solving them as they arise.
- Teaching coping skills, such as strategies to deal with memory difficulties, speech disturbances, fatigue management, movement difficulties.
- Education re: lifestyle modification.

The key components of inpatient multidisciplinary team rehabilitation programmes include:
- A comprehensive multidisciplinary assessment to identify problems which may be improved by input.
- The use of goal setting and action plans to clearly identify the aims of the rehabilitation programme, to establish the wishes and expectations of the person with MS, and to devise a structured plan for addressing these.
- Provision of a wide range of interventions which maximize quality of life by improving functional ability, increasing leisure and work options, and prevent secondary complications (Table 23.4).
- Evaluation of the outcomes of care, typically through measures evaluating function.

Chapter 24

Local services

Inpatient hospital rehabilitation/care

Care within a hospital setting may be required when the person is experiencing an acute episode of neurological symptoms, during which time they often receive a course of high-dose intravenous corticosteroids. Although the majority of relapses resolve completely, up to 40% may leave some residual problems. Therefore while steroids might hasten the role of recovery from a relapse, there is also a role for the multidisciplinary team in helping to manage any residual deficit. There is now evidence available demonstrating that multidisciplinary team intervention provided alongside steroid treatment provides better functional outcomes compared to steroid treatment alone.

The focus of rehabilitation input within this situation is often nursing, physiotherapy and occupational therapy. Typically, rehabilitation interventions focus on providing support both in terms of equipment and personal care; advice and information; and exercise to promote recovery of muscle activity. Occupational therapy is particularly important when home alterations or extra help is required on return home. Access to an orthoptist should also be considered.

At times, bed shortages on neurological wards mean that people are sited on outlying wards within a hospital. This has significant disadvantages. It is not uncommon during these occasions for people with MS to complain that their function actually deteriorates during hospitalization, either because they cannot access appropriate equipment (such as wheelchairs); find the environment is not suited to their individual needs (for example, no grab rails; large spaces to negotiate); or find the help they receive is inappropriate (for example, a lack of staff knowledge about their specific needs; rushing during mealtimes or dressing; inadequate positioning in the bed or chair). Indeed there are many stories of people with MS developing secondary complications such as urinary tract infections, pressure areas and contractures during their hospital stay. This clearly should be avoided at all costs. This may be helped, in part, by staff listening carefully to the person with MS and their family about their needs as well as their thoughts about potential solutions to some of these issues which confront them during their hospitalization. Importantly, where available, specialist MS nurses or therapists should be encouraged to make contact with ward staff and offer advice, information and training, to ensure the person with MS is managed appropriately during their hospital admission. In addition, referral should be made to a specialist neurological rehabilitation service when necessary.

Outpatient rehabilitation services

Local outpatient services may include:
- Physiotherapy
- Occupational and therapy
- Speech and language therapy.

This pathway is often chosen when less intensive input is required, often from a single discipline. Outpatient treatment has the advantage of enabling people to remain at home or in work while participating in therapy interventions. A disadvantage is that it can be very tiring for the person, particularly if travel to and from the appointments is either long or difficult. Fatigue can be particularly problematic in hot weather.

Intervention is usually offered for a finite period, and is designed to achieve specific goals. It is important that the person knows about how to re-contact the service should they require further input at a later stage. Different referral systems exist with some services accepting patient self-referrals, while others require referral from another health professional such as a doctor. This has been explained in some detail in Chapter 22 (Models of care and organization of service delivery).

Community based services

The general practitioner (GP)

The management of MS is primarily the responsibility of the GP in the community, yet each GP in the UK may only have one or two people with MS on their patient list. Ideally, most services should be community-based with supporting expertise from the acute hospital or rehabilitation centre at times of particular need (for example, at diagnosis or at the time of a severe relapse), or complexity (when multiple symptoms interact and intensive inpatient rehabilitation is required). Given the lifelong nature of the disease, the GP is very often the person who sees the person with MS most often, and over the longest period of time. However, because MS is a relatively rare condition for GPs, and they may be unfamiliar with managing many of the problems, it can be extremely daunting for the GP who is required to negotiate the complex network of (often fragmented) services available to people with MS, in order to refer them appropriately.

The community rehabilitation team

Community rehabilitation enables assessment and rehabilitation intervention within the community. The community includes areas such as public transport, workplaces, educational establishments, sports centres and day centres, although it is very often undertaken within the person's home environment. The advantage of this is that the interventions and provision of aids and equipment can be specifically tailored to the environment in which the person operates.

Just as in inpatient rehabilitation, community rehabilitation teams are multidisciplinary in make-up; and effective teamworking and communication is crucial to successful management. Typically community teams provide physiotherapy, occupational therapy, social work, counselling and psychology input, with access to other services such as speech and language therapy, podiatry, and dietetics as needed.

Different models for the delivery of community rehabilitation services exist. Most community rehabilitation teams are generic in their approach, managing people with a broad range of conditions including orthopaedic, rheumatological, respiratory, and neurological conditions. Some community teams however are organized solely around the management of people with disability which is neurological in origin. There are a few specialist community rehabilitation teams throughout the UK who only manage people with MS (refer to Table 24.1 for a description of one such team).

Table 24.1 Case study 4

Community Multiple Sclerosis Team, Regional Neurological Rehabilitation Centre, Newcastle

The Community Multiple Sclerosis Team was established in 1995 to serve the city's population of people with MS. The team was set up as a joint venture between health, social services and the local branch of the MS Society.

The multidisciplinary team is based in the community. It provides physiotherapy, occupational therapy, social work, counselling and psychology input, with access to other services such as speech and language therapy, podiatry, and dietetics. It has developed a referral protocol, a course for people newly diagnosed with MS 'Getting to Grips', an exercise group and a fatigue management course.

It sets itself benchmarks, 'Gold Standards', which were updated in 2003. The team has been awarded the Measuring Success award by the MS Society.

The team has links with MS specialist nurses and neurologists based in the local acute trust to develop joined up local services for people with MS. The team is also a member of the Regional Partnership Forum, an MS Society initiative to improve services for people with MS, which brings together all regional charities, health and social care providers.

Source: *http://www.dh.gov.uk/PolicyAndGuidance/HealthAndSocialCareTopics/LongTerm Conditions/BestPractice/CommunityRehabilitation* Accessed April 2006.

Services provided by charitably funded local branches of the MS Society

Local branches of the MS Society can be a useful resource for providing advice and information. The services available differ between different localities, but typically include:

- The provision of MS Society publications; regular newsletters about local events.
- An annual information event/conferences on some aspect related to MS or living with MS.
- Acting as a specific point of contact for people who are newly diagnosed.
- Providing access to a welfare officer that has received appropriate training.

Some local branches also purchase services such as physiotherapy for their members, which include treatments provided on either a one-to-one and/or group basis.

Long-term support

Introduction

Long-term care services include a continuum of preventive, diagnostic, rehabilitative, therapeutic, supportive, and maintenance services, addressing the health, social, and personal needs of individuals with chronic illnesses and disabilities, and their families. These services may include: health care, home care (personal care assistants), adult day care, respite care, assisted living, nursing home care, transportation assistance, and meals.

People with MS may require long-term care at a much younger age than the general population, but nursing homes usually do not provide an environment where younger individuals can function at their highest level, especially if inappropriately grouped with the elderly. Young Disabled Units are typically better suited to meet the needs of people in these circumstances.

Palliative care

Disability and disease progression

People with MS who develop disability and disease progression face a number of challenges. Issues which are present at the time of minimal impairment, such as role as parent, employment options, and symptom management may become even more complex and challenging. Disease progression is usually associated with loss of abilities, activities and life roles which activates grief and need for adaptation. People may need support to identify new goals and make different plans. The need for support and counselling at this period is as important as counselling at time of diagnosis and should not be ignored. People may be called upon to make important life decisions at a time when they may feel least equipped to do so. Health care professionals should help people plan for problems or limitations so that important decisions can be made with deliberation rather than forced upon at time of crisis.

Management of these areas requires an integrated multidisciplinary approach that aims to reduce limitation in activities, restriction in participations and improve quality of life. The key issues for people with moderate disability have been identified as summarized in Table 25.1 whilst key issues for people with severe disability are summarized in Table 25.2.

Professionals working within neurology, rehabilitation and palliative care need to work closely with primary care staff and care providers, including non-NHS care staff (social care, domiciliary and home care staff), combining their expertise to support people in the advanced stages of long-term neurological conditions, such as MS (The National Service Framework for Long-term Conditions, 2005). The guideline suggests that people should receive a comprehensive range of palliative care services when they need to control symptoms. Services should offer a whole-person approach, sensitive communication, have skills to deal with younger adults, end of life issues, family support, specific neurological symptoms and interventions, and expertise in advance directives. In summary, palliative care takes a 'holistic' approach. Services should offer good symptom control such as pain relief, and meet needs for personal, social, psychological and spiritual support in line with the principles of palliative care.

Palliative care is based on the following principles:
- It affirms life and sees dying as a normal process.
- It provides relief from pain and other distressing symptoms.
- It integrates the psychological and spiritual aspects of a person's care.
- It offers a support system to help people live as actively as possible.

Palliative care models of service interaction acknowledge the need for close coordination whilst recognizing and respecting the different professional roles and potential for overlap between specialities.

Evolving models of care include specialist palliative care teams working alongside specialist neurology and neuro-rehabilitation teams promoting more consistent shared practice. All teams are experienced in symptom control; however, there are some differences in roles, as highlighted in Table 25.3. Some examples of good practice are highlighted in Tables 25.3 and 25.4.

Table 25.1 Key themes for people in moderate disability phase

1. Responsiveness to needs related to significant changes in ability and accrued impairment.
2. Access to and choice of different professional services.
3. Access to multidisciplinary expertise in symptom and disability management and treatment.
4. Communication and co-ordination between service providers and care agencies.
5. Empowerment of person with MS and their carers to enable them to take a partnership role in disease management and treatment.

Source: European Multiple Sclerosis Platform (2004).
Recommendations on rehabilitation services for persons with MS in Europe.

Table 25.2 Key themes for people in severe disability phase

1. Provision of appropriate respite care and short breaks for both the carer and the person with MS.
2. Provision of appropriate long-term facilities.
3. Access to information about services and community care resources.
4. Expertise in caring for persons with MS with severe disability.
5. Coordination of all services.
6. Adequate and appropriate community care services, including home adaptations, mobility equipment and aids, health services.
7. Appropriate palliative care.

Source: European Multiple Sclerosis Platform (2004).
Recommendations on rehabilitation services for persons with MS in Europe.

Table 25.3 Roles of key players in palliative care management

- Neurologists: primary providers of assessment, diagnosis and management of disease.
- Rehabilitation Consultant: primary providers of therapy, equipment, social/psychological support and service coordination.
- Palliative care consultants: providers of terminal care, management of death and bereavement.

Table 25.4 Examples of good practice

St Richard's Hospice in Worcester has appointed a nurse specialist whose remit is to develop specialist palliative care services for people with non-malignant conditions. The post holder hopes to develop the service to provide homecare support in the community. There is strong commitment to developing collaborative working practices with local neurology teams and MS nurse specialists.

University Hospital North Staffordshire Multiple sclerosis nurses working in collaboration with their local palliative day care team at the **Douglas McMillan Hospice** offer a palliative day care service for people with advanced MS. The day care programme includes various complementary therapies, art therapy, networking, support and socialization, as well as spiritual care and respite for carers.

Brambles works closely with the local hospice, **St Catherine's**, to meet the needs of people with complex needs. An education exchange programme is in place. The two day programme is extremely well received by staff and has raised awareness of the skills implicit in each other's jobs whilst improving communication systems.

Source: MS Society (2006). *Examples of good practice*. Available at: *www.mssociety.org.uk*

Symptomatic management

Introduction

The coordinated management of interrelated symptoms in people with MS is key to successful management. Over time, the majority of individuals develop an increasing number and range of symptoms resulting in progressive and complex disability. This poses particular challenges in terms of management since the symptoms tend to interact with each other and, as a consequence, it can be inappropriate to treat one symptom in isolation. For example, the carrying out of clean, intermittent self-catheterization to manage bladder control must take into account the patient's cognitive ability, upper limb dexterity, and lower limb mobility (for example, in terms of available strength, tone and range of movement). Effective implementation of a self-catheterization regime may therefore require input using a number of different approaches including the provision of information, patient education, therapy from a range of disciplines, and drug treatment. Along the same lines, it is also important to appreciate that the treatment of one symptom may worsen another, such as the effects of anti-spasticity or antidepressant agents in people already suffering from severe fatigue. This underlines the necessity of management being undertaken in a coordinated manner, by a team of professionals who possess different skills and who can offer different approaches to solving these interrelated problems. It also highlights the need for careful ongoing evaluation to ensure that the person is benefiting optimally from the interventions undertaken. This is, at least in part, the rationale behind the need for adopting a goal orientated multidisciplinary rehabilitation approach to the ongoing management of individuals.

The commonest symptoms encountered by a cross sectional sample of an MS population in the SouthWest of England is provided in Fig. 26.1. For pragmatic reasons the following section describes each of the symptoms that are experienced by people with MS in turn; the importance of coordinated approach to the management of interrelated symptoms, however, is stressed.

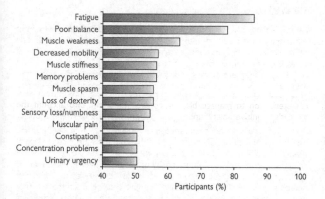

Fig. 26.1 Prevalence of common symptoms in a population of people with MS. Taken from SouthWest Impact of MS (SWIMS) study.

Fatigue

Fatigue is the most common, often very disabling and frustrating, symptom experienced by a person with MS. People with MS rank fatigue as one of the MS-related symptoms that most impairs their quality of life; if severe, it may limit education, employment and social opportunities. The presence of fatigue may vary widely between people with MS and within a person from time to time. It may occur at any stage of the disease trajectory and is often increased at times of relapse.

Fatigue is associated with disability and depression, and it can be difficult to distinguish the impact of fatigue from other symptoms. It is important that health care professionals recognize fatigue when it is present, and assess whether it is a significant problem in a person's life. Assessment of mood, disturbed sleep, and current medications should be made to analyze whether fatigue is primary or symptomatic in nature. Initial therapy for all causes of fatigue should be aimed at optimizing sleep and the person's general daily routine. For example treating nocturnal spasms, nocturia, pain or depression may be enough to establish a normal sleeping pattern and reduce daytime fatigue.

Occupational therapists and/or physiotherapists can be of help in devising personalized fatigue management programmes which include looking at the individual's daily routine to incorporate energy conservation strategies, as well as considering some form of regular exercise, something which has been shown to increase general fitness and reduce fatigue. This may include altering the hours of employment or having a 'nap' after lunch. Some individuals report benefit from drugs such as amantadine or modafinil. Both amantadine and modafinil have been shown in small studies to be of some benefit. Amantadine was originally introduced as an anti-viral agent, but its precise mode of action is uncertain. It is usually used at a dose of 50–100mg twice daily. Modafinil is a more recent drug with a licence for treating excessive daytime sleepiness. It is usually used at a dose of 100–200mg twice daily.

One of the major reasons we do not have good treatments for fatigue is that it is poorly understood as an entity. Although there are many scales purported to measure fatigue, until the concept of fatigue is better understood, the clinical validity of these scales is questionable.

Weakness

Weakness is one of the commonest single symptoms in MS, occurring in up to as many as 85% of people at any time. Lower limb weakness is particularly important since it has been found to be a major determinant of physical functional abilities such as sitting to standing, walking, stair climbing and general mobility. It is noteworthy that a strong relationship has been demonstrated between lower limb weakness and the likelihood of falls.

Clinical issues

Weakness and fatiguability arise primarily as a consequence of demyelination, and secondarily from disuse, especially if the person is sedentary. The range of deficits in weakness vary markedly between individuals and cover the full spectrum from subtle strength and endurance deficits to complete paralysis.

Management

There is now strong evidence to support the use of exercise therapy in improving muscle strength, endurance, and function. Furthermore surveys of people with MS tell us that they consider exercise to be a key element of their overall management, with many people reporting exercise as an area in which they most commonly want advice. The severity of deficits markedly impacts on the different levels and types of activity which an individual can participate in (Fig. 26.2). Early referral to a neurological physiotherapist is therefore important to ensure that specific advice is given and an exercise regimen developed which is appropriate to the individual and their circumstances.

Physiotherapists use a range of interventions to help improve muscle strength and function in individuals. These include:

- Repetition (practise) of functional activities, such as standing up from sitting and stair climbing, using optimal patterns of movement.
- Progressive resistance exercise training, using for example free weights or manual resistance. Studies evaluating the effectiveness of these regimes have demonstrated improvements in muscular endurance, strength and functional performance in tasks such as stair climbing and speed of walking. Importantly these studies have shown that this type of exercise, undertaken 3 times weekly, for periods of 4 to 8 weeks, can be undertaken safely and with no negative effects on fatigue, spasticity, or exacerbation rate. It is generally recommended that these exercise programmes should be designed to activate large working muscle groups in order to avoid overload that results in conduction block when weakness is present. For those with milder deficits in strength, common regimens of strengthening include exercising major muscle groups using weights for approximately 10–12 repetitions through full range of motion for two to three 3 sets, aiming to achieve moderate fatigue by the end of the third set. Exercise programmes need to be progressed according to the ability of the individual, and under the supervision of a neuro-physiotherapist.

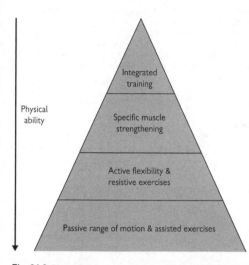

Fig. 26.2 Muscular fitness pyramid. Adapted with permission from Petajan JH and White AT. Recommendations for physical activity in patients with multiple sclerosis. *Sports Medicine* 1999; **27** (3); 179–91.

- Hydrotherapy programmes have also demonstrated to be of benefit in improving muscle strength and endurance. Given the impact that temperature may have on fatigue, a note of caution should be made about ensuring that the water temperature is cooler than that typically used for patients with other conditions, such as arthritis. Temperatures should generally be less than 85°F (29.4° Celsius).
- Home based exercise programmes are another method of enabling people to undertake regular strengthening exercises. Often, use of equipment such as free weights, theraband, or Swiss (gymnastic) balls is used to increase the variety of exercises, in an attempt to maintain interest in, and compliance with, home programmes. Although some studies have demonstrated home programmes to be effective in improving strength and function in the short term, clinical experience suggests that adherence to these programmes over the longer term appears to be poor.

- For some people group exercise classes can be useful in increasing motivation and hence compliance with regular exercise. In part this is probably because of the added social benefits for people. Increasingly group exercise classes are becoming accessible to people with MS, either as a service offered by local physiotherapy departments, or local charitable organisations such as the MS Society groups.
- Links between local leisure centres and neurological physiotherapy departments further increase the range of environments within which people with MS can exercise safely and with confidence.

Spasticity and spasms

Spasticity is a motor disorder which is characterized by an increase in muscle tone and stiffness in response to stretch of relaxed muscle. It is a frequent symptom in MS and is seen, to a greater or lesser extent, in up to 90% of patients at some point in time. Spasticity is usually disabling and can have a major impact on the individual.

Spasticity is one of the cardinal features of the upper motor syndrome, which has both positive and negative features (Table 26.1) which impact on movement. In managing spasticity, it is important to consider the impact of the combination of these symptoms on the impairment of a person's function, since their presence can have a significant influence on the response to treatment.

Terminology

Spasticity has been defined as 'velocity dependent increase in tonic stretch reflexes with exaggerated tendon jerks, resulting from hyperexcitability of the stretch reflex, as one component of the upper motor neurone syndrome hyperreflexia' (Lance 1980). This definition therefore relates specifically to the neural elements of increased tone.

Hypertonus refers to the increased resistance in muscles which arises as a consequence of a combination of both neural (hyperreflexia) and biomechanical factors (adaptive muscle stiffness and soft tissue and muscle contracture).

In practice these terms are often used interchangeably, and, at least in the UK, the term spasticity is the more commonly used term within clinical practice to describe the stiffness which may be felt in muscles as a consequence of an upper motor neuron lesion. Throughout this book the term spasticity will therefore be used to refer to the increased resistance or stiffness of muscles experienced by people with MS, which arises as a consequence of a combination of neural and biomechanical factors.

Clinical presentation

Clinical indications of spasticity are highly variable and may include:

- An increase in deep tendon reflexes.
- An increased responsiveness of muscles to stretch.
- Clonus, a repetitive rhythmic beating movement of a foot or wrist.
- Difficulty initiating movements.
- Impaired voluntary control of muscles.
- Difficulty relaxing muscles once a movement has ceased.
- Sensation of muscle stiffness, tightness or pain.
- Flexion or extension synergy patterns.
- Painful extensor and flexor spasms.
- Decreased range of motion.
- Tendon contractures.

These clinical signs and symptoms may be aggravated by fatigue, stress, urinary tract infections, infections of other origins, and pain.

Table 26.1 Positive and negative features of the UMN syndrome

Negative features	Weakness due to inadequate muscle activation
	Loss of dexterity
	Fatiguability
Positive features	Increased tendon reflexes with radiation
	Clonus
	Spasticity
	Positive Babinski sign (extensor plantar responseS)
	Extensor spasms
	Flexor spasms
	Mass reflex
	Dyssynergic patterns of co-contraction during movement
	Associated reactions and other stereotypical patterns

In MS the lower limbs are usually more markedly affected by spasticity than the arms. From a functional perspective spasticity often impedes mobility, reduces dexterity, and may make it difficult for the patient to remain in a comfortable position, particularly in sitting or lying. Spasms frequently affect activities such as walking, standing and transferring, dressing, personal hygiene, and sexual activity, in terms of quality, independence, and safety. Additionally, spasticity may lead to increased fatigue due to the extra energy expended to overcome tone during voluntary movements involved in activities of daily living. The ongoing presence of spasticity and spasms can also have an emotional impact on an individual, as demonstrated by low mood, poor self-image, and reduced motivation.

Spasticity can sometimes be useful. For example, extensor spasticity of the legs, particularly of the quadriceps, is sometimes advantageous to the patient for standing, walking, and transferring when weakness would not otherwise permit. This is an important point to consider as treatment of spasticity can turn weak stiff legs into weak floppy legs, which may not help the person to walk or transfer.

General principles of management

Spasticity is often poorly managed, and as a result it may be associated with a range of painful and disabling sequelae such as the development of soft tissue contractures and pressure areas. The development of these complications, in turn, often further increases the severity of spasticity and spasms, so that a downward spiral of deterioration occurs. By taking a proactive approach to management, the secondary complications of spasticity, for the most part, are preventable.

Effective management of spasticity and spasm requires a coordinated approach, with the person with MS and their carers closely involved throughout all stages. Close collaboration with members of the multi-disciplinary team, including GP, neurologist, pharmacist, physiotherapist and occupational therapist, is essential.

It is also essential that management of spasticity is always focused on the function and goals of the individual rather than simply aimed at the reduction of spasticity *per se*.

Key components in the management of spasticity include:

- Comprehensive assessment and review.
- The elimination of aggravating factors.
- Patient education and guided self-management.
- Physiotherapy input.
- Pharmacological management.

Referral for specialist advice, for example in multidisciplinary spasticity clinics or specialist seating centres, is sometimes required for individuals with more complex problems (refer to Chapter 23, Specialist regional neurological services for further discussion). These specialist clinics are typically based within or near regional neurological centres.

Spasticity in MS tends to change over time, and it is therefore important to document the evolving impact of spasticity by re-evaluation at regular intervals. This ongoing assessment of change is crucial to enable the appropriate choice and timing of any management strategy.

Multidisciplinary team treatment strategies

There are many strategies available for the management of spasticity. A summary of the decision making processes involved in the management process are outlined in Fig. 26.3.

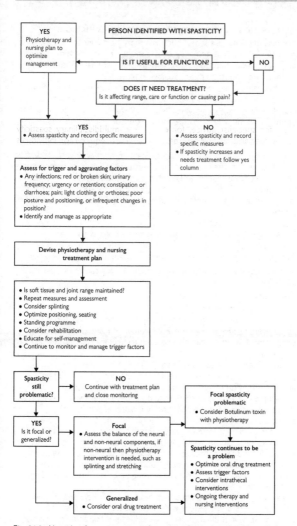

Fig. 26.3 Algorithm for management of spasticity. Reproduced with permission from Thompson AJ. Jarrett L. Marsden J. *et al.*, Clinical management of spasticity (Editorial). *Journal of Neurology, Neurosurgery and Psychiatry* 2005; **76**: 459–63.

Key treatment and management strategies include:

The elimination of noxious stimuli, such as urinary tract infection, constipation, skin irritation or ulceration, ingrown toenails, or tight fitting orthoses. Specific attention is required to diminish or eliminate these prior to commencing or adjusting pharmacological treatment.

Identification of aggravating factors, such as unhelpful compensatory movement patterns (for example pulling strongly into flexion to achieve standing, which may aggravate flexor spasms); poorly fitting splints; adopting positions which may aggravate extensor spasms, such as sleeping in supine.

Education regarding self management of all involved in the care of an individual, regardless of whether the spasticity is mild or severe. This must include the patient, family, carers, and health and social care professionals. Those involved must become knowledgeable about spasticity, its associated features, and how they can avoid trigger factors such as constipation, pain, infections, or poor posture and positioning. Education is particularly important in basic practical issues such as:

- Maintaining good posture.
- Modifying patterns of movement in activities such as transfers.
- Undertaking specific home programmes of activity such as regular stretches, exercises, implementing standing and positioning regimes.

Assistance is often required from family members to achieve this, particularly if spasticity is more severe.

Therapy input

Specific therapy strategies include:

- Maintaining muscle length, through physiotherapy interventions such as passive or active movement and stretching regimens, or standing programmes. Splinting can also be used to maintain or regain muscle length.
- Ensuring close attention is paid to 24-hour management of good posture and alignment by the regular review of positioning regimens and the provision of appropriate wheelchair seating systems.
- Ensuring movement is as efficient and effective as possible through the re-education of movement and of functional activities by physiotherapists and occupational therapists. Short and intensive episodes of therapy, as an inpatient, an outpatient, or within the community setting, can be useful for those experiencing changes in their level of function. Potential areas to be addressed may include mobility functions (such as moving in bed, transfers, walking, using a wheelchair), and general activities of daily living (such as dressing, feeding, and personal hygiene).
- Weakness, which is a negative feature of the UMN syndrome, may be alleviated to some extent with *strengthening exercises* specific to those muscles identified as being weak. General conditioning can also help to strengthen weak and deconditioned muscle groups and increase endurance and cardiovascular conditioning. Strengthening can be achieved in a variety of ways, using free weights, machines, theraband, Swiss balls, or aquatic exercises. Strength training can also assist with the timing of movements, depending on the strength or weakness of the agonist/antagonist muscles.

- The provision of walking aids and equipment is often needed if mobility is difficult (refer to Chapter 29 on mobility for further discussion).
- Functional electrical stimulation can be of benefit in improving gait in selected individuals whose spasticity is relatively mild, but who are experiencing weakness as a predominant symptom of the upper motor neuron syndrome. This requires referral to a neuro-physiotherapist.
- Yoga, t'ai chi and biofeedback may be appropriate relaxation interventions.
- Associated pain may be alleviated or reduced by stretching, transcutaneous electrical nerve stimulation (TENS), or thermal modalities such as cooling. Ergonomic and environmental factors (such as working environment including height of chairs and tables, wheelchair comfort) should also be evaluated as these may be contributing to increased pain.

Pharmacological management

Spasticity can only rarely be managed by antispasticity agents alone. Usually it requires a combination of education, physical therapy and medication. Unfortunately in clinical practice it is not uncommon for medication to be increased before strategies are put in place to eliminate noxious stimuli, identify and address aggravating factors, and instigate an educational programme. It is important to pay attention to all of these factors before resorting to increased pharmacological intervention.

Pharmacological intervention can be divided into:

- Oral therapy (baclofen, tizanidine, benzodiazepines, dantrolene, cannabinoids). Ideally it is better to use one drug on its own, although most of these agents can be used in combination with each other where necessary to improve the clinical effect and lessen side effects.
- Drugs given by other routes: intramuscular (intramuscular botulinum toxin), or intrathecal (intrathecal baclofen or phenol).

Oral drug therapy

Baclofen is often used as a first line drug for management of spasticity. Many people get good to excellent reduction in tone with this medication. It acts as a GABA agonist on the inhibitory GABA-B receptors within the spinal cord, reducing the gain of the stretch reflex loop. The recommended oral dosage ranges from 40–100mg daily. It is started at a low dose of 5mg, two to three times daily and is gradually titrated up to achieve an optimal clinical response with minimal side effects. Although the manufacturer's maximum recommended dose is 100mg daily, many people with MS have been shown to tolerate higher doses. Like all drugs that are used in the treatment of spasticity, baclofen may uncover or exacerbate muscle weakness since it relaxes normal as well as spastic muscles. This can be problematic as patients sometimes rely on their spasticity for support and when it is reduced they find that their limbs are weak and function reduced. Common side effects, particularly at the commencement of treatment, include drowsiness and tiredness, which can be lessened if it is given intrathecally by pump. Nausea, a less common side effect, can usually be avoided by taking baclofen with food. At high doses, baclofen reduces concentration and contributes to fatigue. Overall the drug has a good safety record with long-term use, and the side effects don't build up or become worse over time. If someone is taking high doses of baclofen, the drug should not be stopped abruptly as this may precipitate depression.

Tizanidine is an alpha-2 agonist that decreases presynaptic activity in excitatory interneurones. Its precise mechanism of action is not clearly understood. The results of a number of studies demonstrate that it causes (or uncovers) less muscle weakness than baclofen or diazepam. Tizanidine is usually started at a dose of 2mg twice daily, and increased in 4mg increments every 4 to 7 days to a maximum of 36mg per day, divided into 3 or 4 doses. A common side effect is sedation, and hepatotoxicity may be a problem. Measurement of liver function is therefore recommended before commencement of tizanidine and then regularly after a month of treatment. Other side effects include dry mouth, insomnia, and hypotension. These side effects are dose related and often improve or resolve with a decrease in dosage.

Benzodiazepines (e.g. diazepam, clonazepam) are believed to act on inhibitory GABA-A receptors within the spinal cord. Treatment usually commences with 2mg twice daily of diazepam and is then gradually titrated with 2mg increments up to a maximum dose of 40–60mg per day in divided doses. There tends to be a cumulative effect of diazepam and it may take some time to reach the appropriate levels in body tissues and to reach optimal clinical effect. Benzodiazepines are generally less favoured than baclofen because of their potential to become habit-forming in the longer term, and because of the common side effects that are related to central nervous system depression, and which include drowsiness, sedation, respiratory depression, fatigue, and ataxia. However, for people who are restless or have disturbing night-time spasms, diazepam has the benefit of relieving anxiety and making it easier to relax and get a good night's sleep. Another benzodiazepine, clonazepam, can also help control spasms, particularly at night, but is generally less well tolerated than diazepam due to adverse side effects.

Dantrolene sodium acts peripherally on muscle fibres to produce weakness by inhibiting the release of calcium from the sarcoplasmic reticulum of muscle cells, thereby producing a dissociation of excitation—contraction coupling and diminishing the force of muscle contraction. It is rarely used on its own but may be used in conjunction with baclofen or benzodiazepines. All muscles, both spastic and normal, tend to be affected, ranging from relaxation to weakness, therefore making it less useful for people who walk. The manufacturer's maximum recommended daily dosage in adults is 400mg. The initial dose is typically 25mg per day, which is gradually increased up to 100mg, 4 times per day, according to clinical improvement. If no clinical benefit is noted after 6 weeks, it should be discontinued. Dantrolene commonly causes transient drowsiness, weakness, dizziness and fatigue at the start of therapy but these are generally mild. Muscle weakness can be the key side effect in ambulant people with MS, and it can be particularly problematic in people with pre-existing bulbar or respiratory muscle weakness. Dantrolene can produce serious side effects, including liver damage and blood abnormalities; and the longer the person takes the drug, the more these problems are likely to develop. People taking dantrolene must therefore have periodic blood tests. Dantrolene is generally used only if other drugs—alone or in combination—have been ineffective.

Other drugs used in the systemic treatment of spasticity

Cannabinoids may be useful in the treatment of spasticity and are currently the subject of several clinical trials. At the time of writing, no cannabinoid has a licensed indication for treating spasticity. However, Nabilone (a synthetic cannabinoid) can be prescribed by hospital doctors in the UK and may be useful particularly if there is a combination of pain and spasticity. The usual starting dose is 1mg at night, which can be increased up to 2mg twice daily.

Regardless of the type of medication, to optimize the effectiveness of oral medication, it is important to target treatment at problematic times of the day. For instance, if getting out of bed is difficult following a night's sleep, the medication should be left near the bed so that it can be taken on waking, ideally about 10–20 minutes before getting up.

Intramuscular drug therapy

Botulinum toxin

Botulinum toxin is the most widely used pharmacological treatment to target focal problems with spasticity. The toxin is injected directly into the motor points of the targeted muscle. It takes approximately 10–14 days to have a visible effect. The effect of the toxin is to reduce presynaptic neuromuscular block by preventing release of acetylcholine. Although this blockade is permanent, the nerve sprouting and muscle reinnervation that subsequently occurs means that functional recovery of the muscle occurs within a few months. As a consequence, it may have to be repeated after a few months.

Botulinum toxin is considered to be more useful in the treatment of distal muscles in the arms and legs as the dose of toxin used is relatively small compared to use in proximal lower limb muscles, which require large doses. Injection of botulinum toxin has, however, demonstrated to be useful in the case of severe adductor spasticity, where a reduction in the frequency and severity of spasms together with improvements in the range of hip movement, is associated with improvements in perineal hygiene.

It is essential that botulinum toxin injections are given in conjunction with physiotherapy to optimize benefit.

Intrathecal drug therapy

Intrathecal baclofen

In very severe spasticity, high doses of oral agents are likely to be either ineffective or not well tolerated. When this is the case, intrathecal delivery of the drugs should be considered. The programmable infusion pump is implanted subcutaneously into the abdomen, from where a catheter transports the drug directly into the intrathecal space. Although this is an invasive treatment, which is relatively expensive, it is very efficient since the concentration of GABA receptors in the lumbar spine means that less than one hundredth of the oral dose is required to achieve the required effect, without causing any systemic side effects.

Long-term treatment using intrathecal baclofen has been evaluated and found to be beneficial in carefully selected patients. The selection process should involve consideration both to the functional goals of the patient, as well to their level of commitment in the ongoing maintenance of the pump, which requires regular refills, and replacements on a long-term basis. The administration and coordination of treatment requires specialist input. This type of treatment is most commonly used in people who do not require tone in their legs for standing or transferring. The potential effects are best evaluated by administering a short-acting test dose before a long-term pump is considered.

Common functional goals which may be achieved through the use of intrathecal baclofen include: reducing painful flexor spasms which may awaken patients at night, cause sudden falls in ambulatory patients, or inhibit the ease and safety of hoisting in more severely affected patients; improving hygiene by reducing adductor spasms; enabling the use of orthotic devices; improving bladder and bowel control.

The main complications of intrathecal baclofen pumps are technical. They may include pump malfunction, catheter-related problems (kinking, breaking, displacement), local inflammation, and, very occasionally, spinal meningitis. Programmable pumps tend to cost around £9000 plus the costs of surgery, refilling, and monitoring.

Intrathecal phenol

Phenol is a destructive agent which indiscriminately damages both motor and sensory nerves, and hence it should only be considered in individuals with severe disability who no longer have functional movement in the legs, bowel and bladder function, and in whom sensation in the lower limbs is absent.

Phenol requires administration from a specialist team in carefully selected severely disabled patients. It may be useful in improving aspects of care such as enabling individuals to be seated or to be hoisted safely.

Intrathecal phenol has the advantages of not being as resource intensive as intrathecal baclofen, since the effect of a single injection can last many months and can be repeated if necessary.

Surgical intervention for severe spasticity

On rare occasions, when none of the treatments discussed above have helped, surgery may be recommended for relief in exceptionally difficult cases. The relief is permanent but so is the resulting disability. The techniques used include severing tendons (tendonotomy) or nerve roots (rhizotomy). These measures are only undertaken after serious consideration and for the most difficult cases of spasticity.

Measurement of spasticity

The measurement of spasticity is complex and not well understood. It can be measured through electrophysiological, biomechanical, and clinical evaluation. When evaluating the effectiveness of clinical interventions on spasticity in routine practice it is helpful to complement the neurological assessment with a selection of standardized measures, which may include:

• *Clinician rated measures.* Probably the best known scale is the Ashworth Scale, which is a single item ordinal scale which measures the resistance felt by the rater to passive movement of a limb on a 0 to 4 scale, with zero representing normal muscle tone, and four representing a limb that is fixed in flexion or extension. The Modified Ashworth Scale (Table 26.2) further defines the lower end of the scale by adding the grade 1+. Despite being widely used this scale has relatively limited validity, reliability, and responsiveness data to support its use. Furthermore it does not take into account the impact of spasticity on function.

• *Measures of function,* which are relevant to the person's specific problems, are key to ensuring that measurement of effectiveness remains patient-centred. Some examples include timed walk tests, or recording frequency of falls.

• *Patient self-report measures,* such as visual analogue scales of pain, stiffness, spasm frequency, and severity. Recently, a self-report MS Spasticity Scale has been developed to incorporate the patient experience of spasticity and how it affects people's daily lives. This 88–item, interval-level measurement scale quantifies impact in eight clinically relevant areas: three spasticity specific symptoms (muscle stiffness, pain and discomfort, and muscle spasms), three areas of physical functioning (activities of daily living, walking, body movements), emotional health, and social functioning. Initial evaluation demonstrates it to be a reliable and valid measure of the impact of spasticity. Table 26.3 provides an example of some of the items included within this scale.

Table 26.2 Modified Ashworth Scale for grading spasticity

Grade	Description
0	No increase in muscle tone.
1	Slight increase in muscle tone, manifested by a catch and release or by minimal resistance at the end of the range of motion when the affected part(s) is moved in flexion or extension.
1+	Slight increase in muscle tone, manifested by a catch, followed by minimal resistance throughout the remainder (less than half) of the ROM.
2	More marked increase in muscle tone through most of the ROM, but affected part(s) easily moved.
3	Considerable increase in muscle tone, passive movement difficult.
4	Affected part(s) rigid in flexion or extension.

Table 26.3 The Multiple Sclerosis Spasticity Scale (MSSS-88); some sample items

Section 1. This section concerns muscle stiffness.
As a result of your spasticity, how much in the past two weeks have you been bothered by:

1. Stiffness when walking?

2. Stiffness anywhere in your lower limbs?

3. Stiffness when you are in the same position for a long time?

4. Stiffness first thing in the morning?

5. Tightness anywhere in your lower limbs?

Section 2. This section concerns pain and discomfort.
As a result of your spasticity, how much in the past two weeks have you been bothered by:

13. Feeling restricted and uncomfortable?

14. Feeling uncomfortable sitting for a long time?

15. Painful or uncomfortable spasms?

16. Pain when in the same position for too long?

Section 3. This section concerns muscle spasms.
As a result of your spasticity, how much in the past two weeks have you been bothered by:

22. Spasms that come on unpredictably?

23. Powerful or strong spasms?

24. Spasms when first getting out of bed in the morning?

25. Spasms provoked by changing positions?

Scoring:
Each item is scored on a scale of scale of one to four where: not at all bothered= 1;
a little bothered = 2; moderately bothered= 3; extremely bothered = 4

Developer's reference:
Hobart JC. Riazi A. Thompson AJ. *et al.* Getting the measure of spasticity in multiple sclerosis: the Multiple Sclerosis Spasticity Scale (MSSS-88). *Brain* 2006: **129**; 224–34.
Relevant website:
www.pms.ac.uk/cnrg

Cardiorespiratory fitness

Even in the early stages of the condition, people with MS have been shown to adopt a less active daily routine and are less fit than normal sedentary subjects. This is most likely because of the impact of physical difficulties (however subtle) such as weakness, fatigue, balance problems and spasticity. Historically this situation was actually encouraged by health professionals who believed that exercise (both aerobic and resisted strengthening exercise) was detrimental to people with MS as normal physical and psychological stress would enhance disease activity, and worsen symptoms such as fatigue and spasticity. As a consequence, advice was given to patients to restrict stressful activities and not to undertake vigorous exercise. This perspective has now been turned on its head, and there is now good quality scientific evidence from an increasing number of studies supporting the use of exercise therapy in improving cardiorespiratory fitness in people with MS.

Importantly the evidence shows that there appears to be no deleterious effects of exercise, either with regard to triggering exacerbations, increasing disease activity, or worsening fatigue or spasticity. Indeed avoiding exercise has disadvantages. Sedentary people have an increased risk of developing a large number of other health problems, like obesity and cardiovascular disease. In addition the very low activity levels observed in people with MS often coincides with a loss in leisure activities, social contacts and normal activities of daily living which are important for self esteem and psychological well-being. Reluctance to participate in exercise can result in a downward spiral of inactivity, which has negative physical and psychological consequences for the individual (Fig. 26.4). Exercise should therefore be strongly promoted for people with MS who are not experiencing, or recovering from, an exacerbation. The role of doctors in promoting this is essential since studies have found that one of the most important factors in stimulating involvement in regular physical activity is the referring physician's recommendation to exercise.

Practical issues to consider relating to exercise

The symptoms of MS can make it more difficult for some people with MS to exercise. Even subtle physical or cognitive deficits can mean that people lose confidence in their own abilities to exercise, or may no longer be able to undertake the type of exercise they are familiar with. Referral to a neuro-physiotherapist is therefore important to enable an assessment of the person's individual needs, and for specific advice to be provided about the types of exercise that may be most beneficial for them.

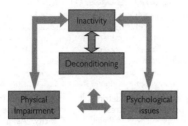

Fig. 26.4 Spiral of inactivity.

Physiotherapists need to consider the interaction of a range of factors when designing exercise programmes. These include:
- Fatigue
- Comfort
- Motivation
- The pattern and severity of disability
- Impairments such as spasticity, weakness and ataxia
- Barriers that can hinder the uptake of exercise opportunities, such as fear, cognitive issues, and difficulties with access such as problems with transportation
- Environmental conditions (such as temperature which should be less than 85°F/29.4°C).

By taking these factors into account, exercise programmes can be developed which are appropriate to the individual's circumstances and level of disability. Physiotherapists can also provide important links to the community by collaborating with local leisure facilities in order to: highlight the specific difficulties an individual may have in undertaking exercise regimens; increase staff awareness of the impact MS can have on the ability to exercise; and provide advice on issues such as whether any equipment would facilitate exercise for an individual.

Aerobic exercise regimens designed to improve cardio-respiratory fitness

Studies demonstrate that aerobic exercise designed to improve cardio-respiratory fitness should ideally be undertaken three or more times per week at a moderate level of perceived exertion (approximately 65% of VO_2 max), for 20–30 minutes, with a 5 minute warm-up and cool-down period. It is recognized that for many individuals a gradual progression to achieve 20–30 minutes is required, and where fatigue is more severe intermittent sessions (for example two sessions of 15 minutes) may be preferable.

Advice to give patients about exercising

- Regular activity is required to make long-term gains, therefore it is important to choose a form of exercise which is enjoyable and can be easily incorporated and sustained into their lifestyle. This might include different forms of exercise such as yoga, t'ai chi, pilates, group aerobic classes, treadmill training, or stationary cycling. While there is currently a lack of studies comparing one form of exercise to another, it would appear from the available evidence that no one specifically targeted exercise programme appears to be significantly more effective than another.
- Start exercising in small amounts, and gradually build up the intensity and duration of the exercise undertaken according to the person's own tolerance.
- Exercise need not only be undertaken in the form of a structured exercise progamme. Incorporating exercise into the normal daily routine is also beneficial to improve general level of fitness. This may include, for example, persevering with activities of daily living such as housework, or stair climbing.
- It is hard to keep motivated to exercise and therefore it can be useful to encourage a partner/friend to join in—this may help not only with motivation, but also with practical issues such as transportation. Setting goals and writing an activity log book can also be helpful motivators.
- Increases in temperature may impact on fatigue, therefore:
  - Ensure the exercise environment is not too hot.
  - Drink cold water before, during and after exercise.
  - Pre-exercise cooling can be beneficial (such as a cool shower).
  - Wear light clothing during the activity.
  - Work at a pace that does not allow overheating.
  - Build in rest breaks as needed; this helps with fatigue and allows the body to cool down.
  - Avoid swimming in heated pools.
- Provide reassurance that it is not uncommon to develop mild neurological symptoms during exercise (such as fatigue, visual and sensory disturbances). These symptoms generally resolve within an hour, or more rapidly with cooling. Individuals should be encouraged to monitor the impact of exercise on any changing symptoms by 'listening to their body'. If symptoms persist they should stop exercising and talk to a health professional about whether/how to adapt the activity so that it can be continued.
- Vigorous exercise should be temporarily discontinued during a relapse or if taking corticosteroid treatment. On recommencement the person should start exercising slowly and monitor how the relapse has affected things.

Further sources of information
- MS Society of Great Britain, *www.mssociety.org.uk*, Keeping Active with MS Factsheet
- MS Trust, *www.mstrust.org.uk*, 'Be Inspired—stay active' CD
- Inclusive Fitness Initiative, *www.inclusivefitness.org.uk*
- Disability Sport England, *www.disabilitysport.org.uk*
- British Wheelchair Sports Foundation, *www.britishwheelchairsports.org*

Ataxia and tremor

Ataxia and tremor occur in approximately 60% of patients with MS. Ataxia is the lack of or reduction in coordination. In MS it is invariably associated with tremor, which is an involuntary, rhythmic, oscillatory movement of a body part. The tremor manifests both on action including posture (postural), during movement (kinetic), or both. In clinical practice it is difficult to disentangle the ataxia and tremor since the tremor is usually embedded within a complex ataxic movement disorder.

Clinical presentation

- The tremor and ataxia is most frequently noticeable in the upper limbs, although it can also occur in the legs, head (titubation) and trunk. They affect upper limb function, gait and balance.
- These symptoms are frequently embarrassing. The typical staggering gait pattern observed is often confused by onlookers as being due to drunkenness. Feeding is also often difficult and messy even when the symptoms may be relatively mild.
- Ataxia and tremor can be severely disabling, and in about 10% of people the symptoms are incapacitating. In severe cases of truncal ataxia, standing and sitting balance can be significantly impaired.

Management

Management of ataxia and tremor is extremely difficult and is typically associated with a poor outcome. Key components of management include:
- Comprehensive assessment and review.
- Multidisciplinary team input with a focus on patient and carer education.
- Pharmacological management.
- Surgical intervention.

Multidisciplinary team input

Referral to occupational therapy and physiotherapy is particularly pertinent. Management strategies include:
- Provision of advice and information re: the use of helpful compensatory strategies to reduce tremor and ataxia, and optimize functional abilities. Upper limb function may be improved, for instance, through techniques such as stabilizing the upper limb by resting the elbow and/or forearm on a table top, or into the side of the trunk. This can be helpful when eating or drinking, when writing or using a computer keyboard.
- Improving posture and proximal stability during activities through postural re-education and strengthening activities.
- Provision of aids and equipment to optimize function such as non-spill cups and straws for drinking, or walking aids such as rollator frames, which increase stability through widening the base of support. Posture and seating equipment, such as a head rest or high backed chair, can be helpful in reducing head titubation. The provision of these relatively simple aids and equipment can dramatically improve a person's quality of life, since they may have a number of benefits such as enabling better visual focus for reading and watching television; and improving head and neck posture, thereby easing swallowing.

Pharmacological intervention

Effective treatment with medication is limited but is worth trying. The most commonly used group of drugs are the beta adrenoceptor blockers such as propranolol. Sometimes high doses may be required if the individual is able to tolerate them (e.g. 180–360mg/day of propranolol). An alternative is primidone, an older barbiturate drug most commonly used to treat epilepsy. This is best started at low doses (around 50mg) and increased if necessary and tolerated, up to 250mg three times a day. Liquid formulations are more amenable to this dose adjustment. Isoniazid (with pyridoxine) has been shown to be of limited benefit in a number of small studies, but practical experience shows it to be less than effective, and it is often not well tolerated. Other drugs, including carbamazepine, clonazepam, buspirone and cannabinoids have been used, although these have been less well evaluated. Alcohol has long been used for treating essential tremor, and sometimes it is worth assessing whether it helps with MS related tremor.

Surgical intervention

Information on the benefits of surgical intervention is gradually accumulating. Surgical intervention is usually considered only in selected patients when ataxia and tremor is very severe and disabling. The two most common options are thalamotomy and deep brain stimulation.

Thalamotomy

There has been limited evaluation of this intervention to relieve tremor in MS. A small number of studies have shown that thalamotomy of the ventral intermediate nucleus alleviates contralateral limb tremor and results in functional improvement, although sometimes this is of a temporary nature. It has been suggested that the zona incerta may be the preferred target, particularly when there is a proximal tremor component. Unfortunately side effects may occur in up to 45% of patients and include hemiparesis, dysphasia, and dysphagia in up to 10% of patients.

Chronic deep brain stimulation

A small number of studies of selected patients have shown that tremor is significantly reduced with thalamic electrostimulation through implanted electrodes. Although serious side effects may occur, presently this is considered to be safer than lesional surgery, particularly for bilateral procedures. Complete cessation of tremor is not necessarily achieved by this procedure. Furthermore tremor control may decrease over time requiring frequent reprogramming. It is not clear whether this is related to underlying disease progression, declining effectiveness of the deep brain stimulation, or both. Nevertheless in those patients in whom the tremor is incapacitating and resistant to conservative management, this procedure may be worthwhile trying. It is particularly worth considering in people where muscle strength is preserved but tremor is disabling.

Measurement of tremor

It is helpful to undertake standardized outcome measures at regular intervals to monitor the severity of the tremor. Methods which are easy to incorporate within clinical practice include:

• Recording specimens of the patient's handwriting.
• Drawing of a spiral.
• Self-report estimates of tremor severity (on a 0–10 rating scale).

Together with standardized assessments of function, these measures are useful in monitoring treatment effectiveness.

Swallowing difficulties (dysphagia)

Difficulty with swallowing (dysphagia) results from any disturbance of the normal process of swallowing. It occurs in approximately 50% of people with MS, often in acute or later stages of disease. Dysphagia can significantly affect an individual's quality of life, since eating and drinking are not purely functional activities but provide an important context for many social interactions. It can therefore have a significant impact on the person both physically and emotionally.

Clinical presentation

Early symptoms include: coughing when eating; pocketing of food in the mouth; hoarse wet sounding voice; frequent throat clearing; anxiety about swallowing; food 'sticking in the throat'; avoidance of certain foods or drinks, and observed weight loss. Such symptoms are often overlooked until the patient has a severe choking episode.

More severe dysphagia can have serious consequences for the individual, including choking or aspiration of food or saliva. Possible signs of aspiration include a wet gurgling quality of the voice; coughing, spluttering, or choking before, during, or after eating or drinking; cyanosis; wheezing; spiking a temperature; increased mucus production and, at worst, chest infection or pneumonia.

In addition to a patient history and physical examination, the diagnosis of dysphagia is established by a speech and language therapist, using a range of investigations which may include videofluoroscopy (barium swallow).

Management

Unfortunately minor swallowing problems are frequently not reported by patients, or detected by clinicians. However early intervention can prevent difficulties later on in the disease, and hence early referral to a speech and language therapist is recommended.

Mild dysphagia is usually relatively easily managed with assessment and advice from a speech and language therapist. This input may include:

- Guidance regarding modification of diet and fluids, such as thickening fluids and avoiding dry or chewy textures. Sticky, solid, crumbly foods or liquids are more difficult to swallow and are therefore more easily aspirated.
- Teaching compensatory postural techniques in an attempt to improve the direction of food flow in the pharynx .
- Teaching of swallowing manoeuvres, such as the use of a double swallow to reduce the residue in the pharynx in order to reduce the risk of aspiration. It is important that the patient actively engages in these manoeuvres and hence they must be cognitively able to understand and follow the instructions.

Drugs can exacerbate dysphagia, either from side effects or from drug action. For example dry mouth (xerostomia), is a common side effect of oxybutynin chloride, which is used to treat neurogenic bladder disorders. Possible strategies include substitution for the drug, use of a saliva substitute, or sips of water between meals.

As swallowing difficulties progress, the problems frequently require multidisciplinary team management. The goal of rehabilitation is to maintain the highest degree of swallowing possible, to prevent or decrease risk of aspiration, and to maintain adequate nutritional status.

Often in MS aspiration may be silent because patients are desensitized to the cough reflex, due to chronic aspiration (chronic laryngeal stimulation). Aspiration pneumonia is potentially serious and so clinicians should always be aware of the potential for dysphagia.

Aspiration and choking as well as the potential development of malnutrition, dehydration and pneumonia may mean that percutaneous gastrostomy (PEG) may be required to ensure intake is safe and adequate. However, the stage of disease progression and other individual factors have to be considered by the person with MS, family and multidisciplinary team before a PEG is deemed to be an appropriate course of action.

Speech difficulties

Dysarthria

Speech disturbance in MS is most commonly due to dysarthria. Dysarthria is a collective name for speech disorders resulting from disturbances in the motor control of speech production. These may include spasticity, weakness and/or poor coordination (ataxia) of the muscles involved in respiration, phonation, nasal resonance and articulation. The prevalence of dysarthria in MS is a matter of some controversy and is dependent on the type of professional assessment performed. Neurologists detect dysarthria in approximately 20% of patients, in contrast to speech and language therapists who detect subtle signs in about half of all patients with MS.

Dysarthria in people with MS is strongly correlated with multiple-system demyelination and disease progression. There are two general causes for speech problems:

- Lesions in the cerebellum: and
- Demyelination in the brainstem affecting the muscles used in speech.

Clinical presentation

Typical speech problems include hypernasality, difficulties with pitch and volume control, and imprecise or poorly coordinated articulation. These difficulties result in reduced intelligibility and speech naturalness.

Management

Management by a speech and language therapist is helpful and should be initiated as soon as possible. It enables a comprehensive assessment of speech production using a range of objective and subjective assessment tools. Therapy interventions should involve both the person with MS and their family. They may include:

- Exercises to help improve speech intelligibility, for example, by reducing rate of speech or improving loudness control.
- Education re: appropriate breathing and phrasing patterns; the use of compensatory strategies such as postural adjustments of the head; and useful communication strategies such as utilizing short sentences.
- Devising alternative communication strategies, such as advice about using gesture to complement speech (for example, shoulder shrugging) and the use of communication aids.

Communication aids may be useful in patients with more severe dysarthria. A range of augmentative and alternative communication aids are available, from low to high tech devices. These may include:

- Head worn voice amplifiers.
- Communication boards to display pictures, or words for basic needs.
- Computerized communication aids with digitally recorded or synthesized speech, utilizing a range of switches or access devices, for example head switches.

Unfortunately, it is often the case that by the time a person with MS requires augmentative and alternative communication aids the usefulness of high tech devices is limited by the severity of concomitant motor, visual and cognitive difficulties.

Dysphasia

The more obvious aphasic syndromes are not commonly present in MS, although language disorders do occasionally occur, usually in patients with more severe cognitive deficits.

Clinical presentation

Individuals suffering from subtle language deficits in verbal expression may express difficulties in conveying their thoughts and needs to others. Although this remains an area of some controversy, it is thought that these language deficits are likely to be a consequence of difficulties with cognitive processing. It is generally agreed that an interdependent relationship between cognition and language exists. Deficits in cognition are therefore likely to directly impact on language and communication. For example, the speaker needs to be able to store events in memory, integrate new and existing knowledge, and retrieve this as necessary in order to communicate. Common language difficulties which are experienced by people with MS include difficulties with naming, word fluency, and sentence comprehension.

Management

To optimize the successfulness of rehabilitation it is important to be aware of subtle language deficits which may exist. Referral to a speech and language therapist may be helpful. The rehabilitation team can also incorporate useful approaches into their programmes such as:

- Providing repetitive or written information to enhance understanding and memory of information and advice given.
- Altering the physical layout of a work space so as to minimize distractions and extraneous noise.

Respiratory difficulties

Respiratory dysfunction is common in people with MS, affecting as many as 70% of people, particularly if the disease is more severe. It is important to recognize as it may be associated with recurrent respiratory infections, particularly if associated with swallowing problems.

Clinical presentation

Restrictive symptoms include reduced vital capacity, inspiratory and expiratory flows; and maximal voluntary ventilation. These are the results of progressive declining motor respiratory muscle weakness (including diaphragmatic weakness) which is required for efficient respiration, as well as poor postural control resulting in the adoption of postures which hinder effective breathing patterns and lung volumes.

Respiratory dysfunction can have a direct impact on speech and may affect sentence length, level, loudness and variability of pitch, and intonation.

Management

Specific respiratory exercises and education re: appropriate breathing patterns can be provided to improve respiratory difficulties. This falls within the remit of both the speech and language therapist and the physiotherapist.

Effective postural management is essential to optimize respiratory function. All members of the multidisciplinary team, within health and social services, as well as the person with MS and their carer, need to take joint responsibility for ensuring effective positioning within the full range of postures adopted by the person.

In an acute event, respiratory support may be required, although this is rare.

Sexual function

Sexual dysfunction is a problem often overlooked by health professionals but is extremely common; in males with MS, the incidence of erectile dysfunction is in the order of 70%. It is usually related to spinal cord involvement and often the occurrence of sexual dysfunction follows on from the development of urinary problems. Apart from erectile dysfunction, failure to achieve orgasm and ejaculatory difficulties may also occur in men. Psychosexual counselling should be considered in all cases alone or in combination with other therapies. The advent of the phosphodi-esterase 5 inhibitors such as sildenafil, tadalafil and vardenafil which are fast acting oral drugs have reduced the need for more invasive techniques such as intracavernosal injection of alphaprostadil (prostaglandin E_1). Sildenafil may be used at an initial dose of 50mg orally before inter-course, and if unsuccessful, then higher doses can be tried.

In addition, impairments such as spasms may make sexual activity difficult which may make it problematic for the person to establish or maintain partnership relations.

Sexual dysfunction may be manifested as loss of libido, loss of vaginal tone, painful heightened vaginal sensation, and loss of ability to orgasm in females. The use of lubricating gels may be helpful and there is some evidence that sildenafil may help some individuals, although the response is less clear than in men.

Health professionals should appreciate the private and intimate nature of discussing sexual function. People with MS should be asked sensitively about, or given the opportunity to remark upon, any difficulties that they may be having in establishing and/or maintaining wanted sexual and personal relationships, and should be offered information about locally available counselling and supportive services. It is deemed good practice to offer every person or couple with persisting sexual dysfunction an opportunity to see a specialist with particular interest in sexual problems associated with neurological disease. Information leaflets with advice on body mapping, lubricants, and the use of sexual aids should be made available.

Pain

Pain in MS is common, with incidence rates reported to be between 28% to 86% of patients. Pain may arise either directly from the neurological damage (neuropathic pain) or from musculoskeletal problems due to reduced mobility. People with MS may also have pain from unrelated causes. Most have chronic pain but an estimated 10% have acute paroxysmal pains, the commonest of which is trigeminal neuralgia, which occurs much more often in MS patients than in the general population. Trigeminal neuralgia is a sharp lancinating pain, radiating down the distribution of the affected branches of the trigeminal nerve. It usually responds fairly well to carbamazepine or gabapentin.

Like many of the commonly used drugs for the treatment of pain and spasticity, there is a large dose range that may be tried. Carbamazepine can cause drowsiness and poor concentration, so is best started at doses of around 50–100mg three times a day. Sometimes people can tolerate doses as high as 600–800mg three times a day, but many people find doses around 200mg three times daily are adequate. Slow release carbamazepine may be useful, often 200–400mg twice daily. Gabapentin has an even larger dose range, and often people with MS require very high doses. The recommendations suggest starting at 300mg at night, and gradually increasing every 2–3 days until pain subsides or side effects occur. Although the manufacturers recommend 800mg three times a day as the maximum dose, sometimes people with MS related pains may tolerate levels up to twice this amount in order to obtain relief.

Trigeminal neuralgia associated with MS can also be treated with interventional procedures such as radiofrequency ablation and stereotactic radiosurgery using gamma knife. These procedures require specialist referral and are performed in few centres.

Other paroxysmal pains also occur, including dysaesthetic burning pains precipitated by touch, movement or hyperventilation. Painful tonic spasms may be associated with these and may be helped by carbamazepine, gabapentin or lamotrigine. Dysaesthetic pain often involves the extremities. This can be very debilitating for the individual, interfering with mobility, sleep, and contributing to depression. The most useful drugs are carbamazepine, gabapentin, pregabalin and the tricyclic antidepressants, particularly amitriptyline. Amitriptyline can cause drowsiness and is best started at a low dose at night (10–20mg), and can be increased as necessary.

Some of the newer antiepileptic drugs including lamotrigine, levetiracetam and oxcarbazepine have also shown some benefit in small trials. Other forms of chronic pain may be secondary to spasticity, or to immobility; back pain is particularly common in wheelchair users. Pain relief should include local measures such as heat pads and transcutaneous electrical nerve stimulation (TENS); although medication such as short-term non-steroidal anti-inflammatory drug use or simple analgesics may be necessary.

Table 26.4 NICE guidelines on pain

- Each professional in contact with a person with MS should ask whether pain is a significant problem for the person, or a contributing factor to their current clinical state.
- All pain, including hypersensitivity and spontaneous sharp pain, suffered by a person with MS should be subject to full clinical diagnosis, including a referral to an appropriate specialist service if needed.

Musculoskeletal pain

- Every person with MS who has musculoskeletal pain secondary to reduced or abnormal movement should be assessed by specialist therapists to assess the potential for alleviation through exercise, passive movement, better seating and other procedures.
- All people with MS with musculoskeletal pain arising from reduced movement and/or abnormal posture not alleviated by non-pharmacological means should be offered appropriate analgesic drugs.
- Every person with MS who has continuing unresolved secondary musculoskeletal pain should be considered for transcutaneous nerve stimulation (TENS) or anti-depressant medication.
- Treatments that should not be used routinely for musculoskeletal pain include ultrasound, low-grade laser treatment, and anti-convulsant drugs.
- Cognitive behavioural and imagery treatment methods should be considered in people with MS who have musculoskeletal pain only if the person has sufficiently well-preserved cognition to participate actively.

Neuropathic pain

- Neuropathic pain, characterized by its sharp and often shooting nature, and any painful hypersensitivity should be treated using anti-convulsants such as carbamazepine or gabapentin or using anti-depressants such as amitriptyline.
- People with MS with neuropathic pain that remains uncontrolled after initial treatments have been tried should be referred to a specialist pain service.

Reproduced with permission from: *The NICE Guidelines for the Management of MS in primary and secondary care, Clinical Guideline 8*, Chapter 6, 2003.

Bladder and bowel dysfunction

Bladder and bowel dysfunction are extremely common in individuals with MS. Estimates of bladder dysfunction are in the order of 75% and bowel dysfunction approximately 50%. Common bladder symptoms are those of frequency, urgency, and nocturia. However, as bladder dysfunction increases, problems of incontinence, retention and urinary tract infections can all occur. Most of these are a result of a combination of detrusor hyper-reflexia (causing urgency and urge incontinence) and sphincter dyssynergia (causing failure to empty, difficult initiating micturition and frequency, with residual volumes predisposing to infection).

Due to the often-mixed aetiology of urinary symptoms it is important to assess bladder emptying by measuring the post micturition residual volume before initiating any therapy; this can be done by either catheterization or trans-abdominal ultrasound. If there is no residual then detrusor hyper-reflexia can be treated with anticholinergic agents such as oxybutynin or tolterodine. The hazard to treating with anticholinergic therapy without prior assessment is that it may precipitate urinary retention or make residual urine volumes worse. The most commonly used drug is oxybutinin, starting at a dose of 2.5–5mg twice daily. The usual potential complications of anticholinergic treatment including dry mouth, constipation and glaucoma may limit its use. Sometimes alternative anticholinergics may be tolerated better, including tolterodine or propiverine.

If nocturia fails to be controlled with anticholinergics the use of desmopressin (DDAVP) delivered by a nasal spray at night can sometimes be useful, although caution must be taken to avoid overdose and potentially dangerous hyponatraemia.

Other potential agents to reduce detrusor hyper-reflexia include intra-vesical capsaicin or botulinum toxin. Two studies of botulinum toxin type A in MS have demonstrated improvements in urodynamic tests, reduction in incontinence rates and beneficial effects on quality of life with no safety concerns.

Detrusor sphincter dyssynergia can be managed using clean, intermittent self-catheterization (CISC). Often by using a combination of CISC and medication, bladder control can be markedly improved. Occasionally control remains poor and an indwelling catheter needs to be considered; if this is long-term a suprapubic catheter is usually preferred.

Cannabis for bladder dysfunction has been assessed in one small open-label study and as part of larger trials for symptom control in MS. Although no significant effects were seen in the larger studies the open-label study demonstrated a significant reduction in frequency, nocturia and incontinence; however total voided volumes also decreased. There were few side effects suggesting cannabis-based medicines may be a useful addition to the current treatment armament, though further trials are awaited.

Bowel dysfunction is less frequent than urinary dysfunction but still affects a significant proportion of people with MS, and can be extremely distressing. Most commonly, individuals complain of constipation and urgency; incontinence is less frequent. Management is more difficult than bladder dysfunction, but the establishment of a routine is important. It is important to identify and treat constipation as early as possible in order to avoid bowel obstruction and overflow that may sometimes occur. People should be made aware of the normal gastro-colic reflex, whereby food entering the stomach triggers increased bowel movement. This reflex should be made use of in daily bowel actions, so that people often find sitting on the toilet for as long as it takes shortly after breakfast can help educate a slow bowel. Often, treatment with oral agents used regularly is necessary (lactulose, senna, movicol) but glycerine suppositories and micro-enemas can be extremely useful. Incontinence often linked to urgency can be helped with loperamide.

Pressure ulcers

A pressure ulcer (decubitus ulcer or pressure sore) is an area of broken skin that is secondary to unrelieved pressure on the skin, often exacerbated by slight trauma, for example, when being moved. They may range from a minor break to very large deep areas. Once present they can be difficult to heal, and can cause worsening of most impairments.

Many people with MS are at high risk of developing pressure ulcers because they may have, for example, limited mobility, impairment of sensory functioning, and reduced cognitive function. Most pressure ulcers can be avoided by good anticipatory management.

In the NICE guidelines the development of a pressure sore is classified as a sentinel event that needs to be reported. The guidelines provide clear guidance for the prevention and management of pressure ulcers (Table 26.5).

Table 26.5 NICE guidelines for the management of pressure ulcers

Every person with MS who has reduced mobility sufficient to require the use of a wheelchair should be assessed for their risk of developing a pressure ulcer, and should be informed of this and offered appropriate advice.

Every person with MS using a wheelchair daily should be assessed individually by a suitably trained person for pressure relieving devices and procedures whenever admitted to hospital for whatever reason. The assessment should be clinical, specifically taking into account the risk features associated with MS, and not simply the recording of a pressure ulcer risk score, and this should lead to the development and documentation of an action plan to minimise risk including:

• optimization of nutritional status

• provision of suitable equipment

• documentation of agreed manual handling techniques.

Every person with MS provided with a wheelchair by a statutory organization (NHS or social services) or whose wheelchair seating is being reassessed should specifically be considered for pressure relieving procedures and devices not only in the wheelchair but in all other activities, especially transfers and sleeping.

For every person with MS considered to be at risk on their bed (in hospital or in the community):

• An appropriate specialist mattress should be provided wherever they are lying down.

• Regular turning should not be depended upon as a policy for preventing pressure ulcers.

• The skin areas at risk should be inspected to ensure adequate protection is occurring.

If a pressure ulcer occurs, it should be considered an adverse event worthy of investigation and advice sought from a specialist service.

Any person with MS who develops a pressure ulcer should be nursed on a low-loss mattress (while in bed) and the ulcer should be dressed according to appropriate local guidelines.

Reproduced with permission from: *The NICE Guidelines for the Management of MS in primary and secondary care, Clinical Guideline 8*, Chapter 6, p128–9, 2003.

Contractures

Joint contractures occur when the muscle and connective tissue surrounding a joint become shorter and stiffer, resulting in increased resistance to stretch and a reduced range of movement. Severe contractures are not only painful but can limit the person's ability to self-care and make all care very difficult. The primary aim is to prevent contractures occurring, and the most widely used treatment is stretching. Stretching leads to improvement in tissue extensibility; when the stretch is held for a period of time and repeated regularly, the deformation results in permanent lengthening of the muscle fibre and increased flexibility of the muscle and connectivity tissue.

Another method of reducing contractures is serial casting which requires a plaster cast to be applied to the affected joint to maintain the joint in a stretched position. The cast is left on for a period of time, then removed, the joint stretched further, and a new cast applied. Serial casting has been described as effective in improving passive range of movement; however, the disadvantage of the technique is that it requires multiple casting changes. The application of adjustable splints which allow the joint to be fixed with the soft tissues in a lengthened position may prove an advantageous treatment method. The NICE Guidelines provide clear guidance for the prevention and management of contractures (Table 26.6).

Table 26.6 Management of contractures at joints

- Any person with MS with weakness and/or spasticity sufficient to limit the regular daily range of movement around a joint should be considered at risk of developing a contracture at that joint, and should be considered for preventative measures.
- Any person with MS at risk of developing contractures should have the underlying impairments assessed and ameliorated if possible.
- Any person with MS at risk of developing contractures should be informed, and they and/or their carers should be taught how to undertake preventative measures such as regular passive stretching of the joint(s) at risk and appropriate positioning of limbs at rest. In more severe instances, specialist advice should be obtained on seating and positioning, including positioning in bed.
- Any person with MS who develops a contracture should be assessed by a suitable specialist for specific treatment, and the assessment should take into account the problems caused by the contracture, the discomfort and risk of any treatment, as well as the wishes of the person with MS. At the same time renewed efforts should be made to reduce the underlying causes and to prevent further contracture.
- Specific treatment modalities to be considered should include prolonged stretching using:
  - Serial plaster casts or other similar methods such as standing in a standing frame.
  - Removable splints.

These are usually combined with: local botulinum toxin injection, and surgery as necessary.

Reproduced with permission from: *The NICE Guidelines for the Management of MS in primary and secondary care, Clinical Guideline 8*, Chapter 6, p.107, 2003.

Cognitive problems

Cognitive dysfunction can be a prominent feature in MS where it is unrelated to disease duration or to level of physical disability. The prevalence has been reported to be in the order of 54–65% in hospital-based studies, and 40% in a large community-based study. The pattern of cognitive decline in MS is predominantly sub-cortical, with the main deficits being in short-term memory, attention, conceptual reasoning, and speed of processing.

Cognitive impairment can have a devastating impact on psychosocial functioning, for example 50–80% of people with MS are unemployed within 10 years of disease onset despite lower than expected levels of physical disability to explain this. By identifying and assessing the nature and extent of cognitive deficits, appropriate strategies to minimize the impact can be developed.

Assessment by a neuropsychologist is useful in defining the extent of any dysfunction in domains including memory, attention, speed of processing, language, and executive function. Once assessment is complete targeted cognitive rehabilitation programmes can be tailored to the individual and if appropriate in conjunction with their employer.

Mood and emotional issues

Living with MS poses a number of challenges that can affect the way a person feels about themselves (Table 26.7). It is not uncommon for people with MS to experience uncertainty, anxiety, poor self image, and feelings of grief and stress. Health professionals can help support people with MS by providing support and education within an empowerment model so that the person gains a sense of control and is able to participate actively in healthcare decisions and self-management strategies.

People may experience a number of reactions at time of diagnosis. The most common responses include: shock, denial, anxiety, anger, relief. Ongoing emotional reactions include feelings of grief, anxiety, resentment, and guilt.

A number of emotional changes may occur in MS. Mood swings may include emotional lability, and uncontrollable laughter or crying may occur which do not reflect the person's underlying mood. Such pathological laughing or crying may be associated with lesions in the limbic system or related structures. Treatment may include the use of amityriptyline or selective serotonin reuptake inhibitors.

Depression and anxiety respond well to appropriate treatment; however, they are often not assessed. Reported rates of depression range from 10–57% whilst rates of anxiety have been reported at 25%. Depression is more common among people with MS than in other disabling conditions. Possible causes include: disease activity, lesion site, reaction to life changes, and side effects of medications. Suicide is more common among people with MS than both the general population and patients with other neurological conditions. Depression in MS is treated most effectively with a combination of psychotherapy and antidepressant medication. Anxiety responds well to cognitive behavioural therapy programmes.

Table 26.7 Challenges of daily life with MS

- Living with uncertainty
- Being informed—in charge
- Making personal decisions
- Balancing hope and realistic expectations
- Dealing with stress.

Adapted from: Strittamer R. Emotion–related issues of the newly diagnosed *MS in focus*, 2004; 4: 7–9.

Chapter 27

Psychosocial issues

Pregnancy

The effect of pregnancy on disease activity is an important concern among young women. A prospective study of pregnancy in MS confirmed that relapse rate declines during pregnancy, especially in the third trimester, increases during the first three months post-partum, and then returns to pre-pregnancy rate. In the same study epidural analgesia and breast feeding did not increase the risk of relapse. There is therefore no medical contraindication to pregnancy in MS. Women should be encouraged to seek medical advice before conception in order to review any medications and make changes as necessary. None of the disease modifying drugs are considered safe during pregnancy and should be stopped, ideally in advance of conception. Disease modifying drugs may be restarted following delivery if the mother does not plan to breastfeed, otherwise treatment can be resumed once breastfeeding is stopped. There are no contraindications to using analgesia including transcutaneous nerve stimulation or epidural pain relief during child birth.

Vocational activities

People with MS are often well educated and skilled workers with extensive employment histories who constitute a valuable labour resource for the societies in which they live. At diagnosis most people with MS are in full-time education or employment although many subsequently leave work. A recent audit report from a large UK Neurology centre demonstrated that most people with MS are in employment at diagnosis, but that employment loss starts shortly after diagnosis with 80% of people with MS unemployed within ten years of diagnosis. The reasons for unemployment have not been clearly delineated and may be related to the disease itself, or to the working environment and demands of the job.

The need to integrate health and employment teams to improve vocational rehabilitation is now well recognized. In the UK, key documents highlight that people with long term neurological conditions should have access to appropriate vocational assessment, rehabilitation and ongoing support to enable them to find, regain, or remain in work, and access other occupational and educational opportunities. Rehabilitation teams should offer services that provide mechanisms for people with MS to make adjustments in their careers and to continue working as long as they wish to. Good vocational rehabilitation should ideally blend the expertise of health professionals, psychology, counselling, social work, technology, human resources, and law. Early intervention is key to support and train people to enable them to obtain, maintain, and advance in jobs that are compatible with their interests, abilities, and experience.

MS is covered by the Disability Discrimination Act (DDA) from the point of diagnosis in many countries. In the UK, the DDA prohibits unlawful discrimination in all aspects of employment—in recruitment, selection, training promotion, redundancy and dismissal and places a duty on employers to make reasonable adjustments to the workplace or working arrangements (Table 27.1). In the UK an Access to Work scheme is available through disability employment advisors at Job Centre Plus offices who can offer advice re: adjustments, grants, and physical adaptations.

Table 27.1 Reasonable adjustments to facilitate employment

- Allocating some of your work to someone else.
- Transferring you to another post or another place of work.
- Making adjustments to the buildings where you work.
- Being flexible about your hours—allowing you to have different core working hours and to be away from the office for assessment, treatment or rehabilitation.
- Providing training.
- Providing modified equipment.
- Making instructions and manuals more accessible.
- Providing a reader or interpreter.

Adapted from: www.direct.gov.uk

Family issues

MS has been described as 'the uninvited guest' in family life. The unpredictable nature of the disease means that people with MS and their family
members face many challenges in planning and anticipating daily activities.
This can impact significantly on a family's rhythm of carrying out daily
routines and may disrupt communication between family members.

Creativity and flexibility are often required to distribute the resources
of time, energy and emotions appropriately among all family members.
The person with MS and their family may experience feelings of loss
and grief with every new symptom and change in functional ability. Furthermore, people with MS may have difficulty describing unseen silent
symptoms whilst family members may become overprotective, resulting
in unexpressed feelings. Health care teams should be aware of the impact
of MS on family dynamics and should not overlook these issues when
making assessments. It is important that they employ sensitive, skilful
assessment techniques of key areas (Table 27.2), ensuring appropriate
referral to available resources. Useful sources of help and advice are
highlighted in Chapter 32 (Useful Resources).

Telling others

When a person is diagnosed with MS, partners, children, parents, siblings,
extended family, and friends may all be affected. One of the first
questions people may face is whether or not to tell others. The decision
to tell or not to tell is a personal decision that may be influenced by
whether the disease is obvious or not.

People who are obviously affected by their MS symptoms usually find it
useful to talk openly with their immediate family about the diagnosis and
impact of MS. It is important that the person with MS feels adequately
educated and informed to lead discussions. It may be useful to do this
in partnership with a health professional, perhaps arranging a family
appointment with an MS nurse, who can help explain symptoms and
short-term and long-term prognosis. In addition expert patient and expert
carer programmes may help.

Adjustment

The arrival of MS in the family requires a family to make adjustments.
Both the person diagnosed and their family will have to find the best way
of managing and treating MS and how to deal with any future problems
associated with the illness. Family members, for instance, need to learn
how to deal with the fluctuating nature of *attacks*.

One of the biggest challenges a person with MS may face is achieving the balance between independence and the need for support. It is important that health and social professionals raise and discuss this with individuals and families so that they can explore values and agree ways of working together. When talking with the family about these issues it is important to clarify what help is needed, what the person with MS is willing to accept, and what the family (or others) can provide. It is also helpful to try to gauge the need for dependency on others. In some cases family members may try to do too much even when help is not needed, which can create an unnecessary level of dependence. In other cases there can be a reluctance of the person with MS to accept help, which can lead family members to feel rejected and inadequate.

Table 27.2 Assessment of family issues

- Assess family support system.
- Assess family understanding and knowledge of MS.
- Assess family coping behaviours and problem solving techniques.
- Assess impact of MS on parental role.
- Assess impact of caring role on children.
- Assess family activities and financial resources.
- Assess impact and perceived impact of MS on family roles.
- Assess family interactions and communication including expression of emotions.
- Assess need to refer to appropriate support resources.

(Adapted from Springer RA, *et al.* (2001). Psychosocial implications of multiple sclerosis. In *Advanced Concepts in Multiple Sclerosis Nursing Care* (J.Halper, ed) pp. 213–37.

Children

Parents frequently try to protect their children by not telling them anything, especially if there are few physical symptoms evident, believing that their own worries and anxieties do not show. There is now evidence that a parent's level of 'invisible' symptoms of mood and anxiety impact negatively on children. Lack of open discussion can cause uncertainty and fear and may also discourage children from asking questions and talking about matters important to them. By contrast, open communication encourages honesty, and a shared approach to facing the challenges as a family can help the child to cope. Teenagers are at risk of taking on too much care and too many practical responsibilities. Health professionals should be aware of this encouraging use of resources to support and minimize burden. The delivery of educational programme models such as 'MS in the Family' workshops can help facilitate discussion and open channels of communication providing a safe environment for children to share their concerns and learn from each other. Table 27.3 highlights some helpful advice on how to help children to understand MS. Useful sources of help and advice are also highlighted in Chapter 32 (Useful resources).

Table 27.3 Helping children understand MS

Generally, children are less fragile than might be thought, and are capable of coping with stressful events as long as they understand what is happening at their own level, and they feel the problem is being dealt with.

Parents should not try to protect children by hiding MS, but rather engage in open and honest communication about the condition; what it means for them; and how it will affect them and the family as a whole.

Overall it may be useful to talk to children about MS in the context of their life, and that of the family. Try to ensure that it does not become the overriding focus of family life but another factor to consider

How children may feel

Children of any age may worry that their parent may die, and older children may worry that they may get MS themselves. It is useful to provide appropriate information when such concerns are aired and MS teams should explore how best to facilitate this.

Children may feel frustrated if a parent is unable to participate in activities or make commitments the way other parents can.

Some children may also feel ashamed and embarrassed if a parent uses a stick or wheelchair. A discussion about these issues from the perspective of the parent with MS may help clarify things.

It is important that children are encouraged to ask questions. It is also important that parents ask them about their thoughts in an effort to allay some of their concerns.

Answering children's questions

In answering children's questions, it is important to take into consideration the child's age, intelligence and maturity and ensure that they do not feel overwhelmed with information they won't understand, or necessarily need to know.

Generally, children under 4 do not have the capacity to comprehend the implications of MS in the family. These children are influenced by changes in their every day life and respond positively to physical contact and care.

Children from 4 upwards may benefit from brief simple explanations.

Children from 6 upwards may feel insecure about their role in the family and should be made feel cared for and may also benefit from helping with simple child appropriate practical chores to feel useful.

Teenagers often fall into the trap of a caring role. It is important that they are encouraged to engage in their own life and are supported to prevent excessive burden.

If there is more than one child it may be useful to sit them down at different times and talk to them; this will allow you to address them at their level, and answer their own specific concerns and questions.

Adapted from Nabe-Nielsen, M. (2004). How to encourage your children to talk about MS. *MS in focus*, Issue 3.

MS and partners

MS can have an effect on partnership and relationships and can add pressure and strain, as a couple living with MS brings an added element of uncertainty into life together. Joint projects and plans may have to change, and joint wishes may have to be adapted. Many couples review their financial status, and how this affects both short-term and long-term planning. Couples may find that roles and income sources change. Often the partner with MS may decide to leave or change employment without seeking appropriate advice. An assessment by an occupational therapist can be useful to help the person explore employment options. A person's sex life may be affected by MS and couples may need to explore new forms of intimacy. It is important that couples face up to the life changes that MS may bring, and to talk openly with each other. If this is difficult, advice from a marital guidance or family counsellor may prove useful.

Carers

In the UK, a carer has been described by the Department of Health as a relative or friend providing support to someone who in turn needs support because of age, physical or learning disability or illness, including mental illness. There are 6 million carers in the UK and 2.3 million people become carers each year. However, less than a third are assessed by Social Services and some £660 million carer benefits go unclaimed.

In general carers are people who help with the physical, emotional, and daily needs of people who cannot manage all these activities on their own. While some carers are paid professionals, many are family members who provide emotional support, help with daily tasks, chores, and intimate help. Many family members adjust very well to the caring role; however, there is evidence that caring can have a detrimental impact on a carer's psychological well being. A detrimental impact on the psychological well-being status of partners and carers has been demonstrated in a number of studies, and it is therefore crucial that this is acknowledged and addressed by health and social care professionals.

Carers' rights are protected by the Carers [Equal Opportunities] Act 2004 (Table 27.4) which promotes cooperation between authorities. It requires organizations to inform carers of their right to an assessment which takes into account their outside interests such as work, study and leisure. Carers are now entitled to:
- Have a carer's assessment.
- Explore how they feel about caring with a professional.
- Discuss information on benefits and support such as carers groups.
- Decide if they want to stay or return to work and how to make this happen.
- Look at how caring may affect them in the future and what help might be needed.

Despite this legislation studies have shown that care givers experience low levels of perceived social support and have a low uptake of formal community support services.

One of the biggest conflicts that carers face is the need to work in order to meet essential family needs. This frequently results in frustration, exhaustion, and burn out. Carers themselves have voiced some of their main concerns as being:
- Difficulty in accessing information on the illness, the support services available, and how to access information on benefits.
- Poor co-ordination between health teams, and health and social care teams.

Ten practical ways to address these issues, and to support carers include:
1. Listening to the voice of carers.
2. Ensuring the carer has information on the illness, available support services, and is signposted to sources such as benefits information.
3. Ensuring that there are sufficient support services in place on discharge.

4. Giving sufficient notice of, and being flexible about, the timing of the discharge.
5. Ensuring that the patient is not discharged too soon.
6. Improving coordination between health and social care, and between departments within the NHS.
7. Ensuring that vital equipment is available at the point of hospital discharge.
8. Not assuming the carer can cope, give a choice.
9. Ensuring that there is one point of contact.
10. Improving the transport arrangements from hospital.

Useful sources of help and advice are highlighted in Chapter 32 (Useful resources).

Table 27.4 The Carers (Equal Opportunities) Act 2004

- *Clause 1*: gives carers more choice and better opportunities to lead a more fulfilling life by ensuring that carers receive information about their rights to an assessment under the 2004 Act.

- *Clause 2*: ensures that those assessments now consider the carer's wishes in relation to leisure, training, and work activities.

- *Clause 3*: provides for cooperation between local authorities and other public authorities, including housing, education, transport and health, in relation to the planning and provision of services that may help support the carer in their caring role.

Chapter 28

Complementary and alternative therapies

The term 'complementary and alternative therapies' refers to a broad and complex combination of interventions and is also interchangeably called holistic, unorthodox, unconventional, natural, traditional or non traditional, according to your cultural beliefs.

Complementary therapies appear to be widely used by people with MS although their potential benefits in the treatment of MS remain controversial, not least because conclusive evidence about the effectiveness and safety of most forms of complementary therapy is not available.

Bowling[1] reported that the most common reason reported for using complementary therapies was to improve general health. Other reported reasons included attempts to:
- Control symptoms
- Control emotions
- Alter the course of the disease.

Some of the complementary products most frequently used in MS include:
- Bee pollen
- Cannabis/marijuana
- Coenzyme Q_{10}
- Cranberry
- Evening primrose oil
- Flaxseed oil
- Garlic
- Ginseng
- Ginkgo biloba
- Grape seed extract
- Kava-kava
- St. John's wort
- Vitamin B complex.

Other therapeutic approaches used in MS are:
- Acupuncture
- Aromatherapy
- Chiropractic/osteopathy
- Guided imagery and visualization
- Homeopathy
- Hyperbaric oxygen
- Hypnotherapy
- Magnetic therapy
- Massage
- Meditation
- Reflexology
- Reiki
- T'ai chi/yoga.

1 Bowling AC. *Alternative Medicine and Multiple Sclerosis*. New York: Demos Medical Publishing 2001.

Many people with MS try unlicensed therapies in an attempt to self-manage their illness. The rationale for treatment may not exist and placebo effects may occur. In recognition of the fact that many people with MS will explore complementary therapies, NICE guidelines have reviewed the evidence for use and made a number of recommendations (Table 28.1). The recommendations are based on the principle that people should have a choice to pursue treatments they wish, are given information on treatments available, consider the risks, costs, benefits of treatments, whilst keeping health professionals informed of treatments used.

Table 28.1 NICE guidelines on complementary and alternative therapies

A person with MS should be informed that there is some evidence to show benefit for the following but insufficient evidence available to give a more firm recommendation:

- reflexology and massage
- fish oils
- magnetic field therapy
- neural therapy
- massage plus body work
- t'ai chi
- multi-modal therapy.

A person with MS who wishes to consider or try an alternative therapy should be recommended to evaluate any alternative therapy themselves, including the risks and the costs (financial and inconvenience).

A person with MS should be encouraged to discuss any alternative treatments they are considering, and to inform their doctors and other professionals involved of any they are using.

Reproduced with permission from: *The NICE Guidelines for the Management of MS in primary and secondary care, Clinical Guideline 8*, Chapter 6, p132, 2003.

Mobility issues

Introduction

People with MS commonly experience restrictions in mobility. Surveys indicate that as many as 87% of people report difficulties in walking to some extent. Natural history studies show that approximately 50% of people require the use of a walking aid within 15 years of diagnosis, and that this rises to approximately 80% by 30 years post onset. In the progressive form of MS this rate of progression appears to be faster, with 50% of people requiring a walking aid within just 5 years following diagnosis. The evidence demonstrates that mobility limitations are associated with a poorer quality of life; with many people unable to obtain wheelchair access to the places they want to go, and/or having adequate transport facilities to enable them to participate in family, social, vocational, and leisure activities. This can leave people isolated and lonely at home. Assessment and interventions related to improving mobility are therefore a key part of intervention.

Mobility difficulties do not simply relate to problems with walking. Assessment of mobility should be viewed in its broadest perspective and should include aspects such as bed mobility, transfers, walking indoors and outdoors, and community mobility. Comprehensive multidisciplinary assessment and management is therefore required, not only because of the breadth of difficulties faced, but also because the causes of these mobility problems are often multi-factorial and complex in nature. Moreover they cover the whole spectrum of impairments, activities and participations, and evolve throughout the course of the disease (Table 29.1). Attempts to treat one symptom or problem without taking into account others is unlikely to be successful.

Broadly speaking, problems with mobility and balance can be addressed by intervening at the level of the impairment, the restricted activity (disability), or at broader environmental factors. Numerous strategies are available at each level of input. While treatment at just one level is sometimes adequate to solve the problem(s), it is more common for intervention to be required across all levels.

Table 29.1 Common causes of mobility problems

Causes	Examples
Physical impairments	Lower limb and trunk weakness
	Spasticity
	Cerebellar ataxia
	Fatigue
	Altered sensation
	Visual symptoms
	Deconditioning.
Psychological and cognitive issues	Loss of confidence
	Anxiety or fear
	Altered mood, such as depression
	Cognitive impairments such as reduced attention and concentration, lack of insight impacting on safety awareness.
Environmental	Home setup, including access issues such as width of doorways
	Climate
	Outdoor terrain
	Physical barriers such as stairs, or availability of equipment.
Sociocultural	Policies which address the physical and attitudinal barriers confronted by disabled people in different environments; accessible public transportation, accessible accommodation
Economic	The inability of a service (or an individual) to purchase and maintain appropriate equipment, or to modify home and work environments

Multi-disciplinary therapy interventions

A limited number of studies have specifically evaluated the effectiveness of physiotherapy in improving mobility. The evidence demonstrates improved outcomes, at least in the short-term, in relation to the speed and quality of walking, and in measures of balance and general mobility. Neither the method of service delivery (outpatient or community based), or the approach used (impairment based or task oriented) appears to make a difference in terms of outcome. Studies have also been undertaken evaluating the effectiveness of the multidisciplinary package of rehabilitation on a range of daily activities, which included measures of mobility. These consistently demonstrate that aspects of mobility, which include walking and transfers benefit from rehabilitation, delivered in a range of settings. These results have informed the recommendations made in the current national clinical guidelines for MS which state that 'any person whose activities are affected or threatened by reduced mobility should be assessed by a neurology service'; and that 'physiotherapy aimed at improving mobility should be offered to all those whose who are, or who could be, walking'.

A broad range of interventions are used by physiotherapists, occupational therapists and other members of the multidisciplinary team, such as podiatrists, to improve various aspects of mobility. These include:

Identifying and treating any underlying impairments such as weakness, fatigue, spasticity, ataxia, and soft tissue tightness. This includes the prevention of secondary complications which have a direct and negative impact on mobility. Interventions include:
- Implementing a self-stretching and positioning regimen as early as possible. Soft tissue tightness and joint stiffness of the trunk and lower limbs often develops in an insidious fashion alongside deterioration in mobility.
- Strengthening exercises for weak muscles. This may include the use of repetitive resisted exercises, as well as functionally biased activities such as stair climbing or sit to stand.
- Functional electrical stimulation (FES) can be immediately effective in improving foot drop due to weakness and or fatigue. It has also demonstrated to be beneficial in reducing the energy costs of walking. The Odstock dropped foot stimulator (Fig. 29.1) is a single channel foot switch-triggered portable neuromuscular stimulator designed to elicit dorsiflexion and eversion of the foot, by stimulation of the common peroneal nerve (maximum amplitude 100mA, 350mcs pulse, 40Hz). Skin surface electrodes are placed, typically over the common peroneal nerve as it passes over the head of the fibula and the motor point of tibialis anterior. A 2 channel stimulator can alternatively be used for the correction of bilateral foot drop controlled by a single foot switch which times the stimulation to walking. By stimulating dorsiflexion and eversion, the foot clears the ground in the swing phase more easily, thus reducing the effort of walking and reducing compensatory strategies such as hip hitching and circumduction.

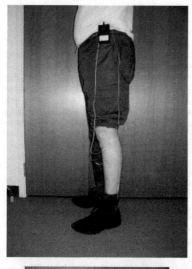

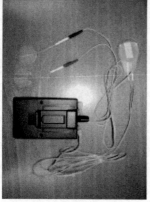

Fig. 29.1 The Odstock dropped foot stimulator.

An immediate benefit of the stimulator is that walking is easier and safer, thereby improving confidence with mobility. In the longer-term, repeated use of the stimulator may lead to a more normal pattern of walking being relearned. A referral to physiotherapy or to a specialist FES clinic is required to determine potential benefits for each individual (refer to Chapter 23, Specialist regional neurological services). Comprehensive downloadable information about FES is freely available for both clinicians and patients at *http://www.salisburyfes.com*

- Programmes aimed at improving cardiorespiratory fitness. These aim to prevent deconditioning, which may further accelerate deterioration in mobility as a result of increased fatigue, weakness, and reduced endurance.

Task-related practice of specific mobility activities. This is typically the remit of the physiotherapist, working in collaboration with other members of the team such as nursing staff and occupational therapists. Task related practice is relevant to the whole gamut of mobility activities including walking (through gait re-education), getting up and down from sitting to standing, transferring to and from a range of surfaces such as bed to chair or wheelchair, toilet transfers, bath transfers, moving within the bed, getting up from the floor, climbing stairs, and manouvering wheelchairs.

Education of more efficient movement patterns to reduce overall levels of effort with mobility tasks. This usually involves teaching the person how to use more efficient patterns of movement and how to minimize and, wherever possible, stop using abnormal movement patterns. When impairments are more severe it includes teaching the person helpful compensatory strategies to optimize their function.

Modification of the environment and provision of equipment. This is usually undertaken by an occupational therapist or physiotherapist. The key aims are typically to increase independence and to reduce the level of effort required for mobility. For example bed levers can be helpful in assisting the person when rolling over or getting out of bed, and raising the height of a chair or bed can reduce the effort of moving from sitting to standing.

Provision of walking aids by a neurological physiotherapist with the aim of improving safety, efficiency and quality of walking. A wide range of walking aids is available, and therefore individual assessment of need is required.

Implementation of standing regimens

One of the most difficult phases of management is when people are standing and walking less and are spending an increasing amount of time in a wheelchair. At this stage it often difficult for people to exercise safely and effectively. The implementation of standing regimens, through the use of standing frames such as the Oswestry standing frame, can be a useful intervention during this phase.

Standing regimes can be implemented on a daily basis within a person's home setting as part of an overall management programme. Generally this can be achieved for periods of approximately 30 minutes (a graduated programme may be necessary to achieve this initially). Although there is little scientific evidence to substantiate its impact, the prolonged weight bearing, combined with good alignment of joints and soft tissues, is believed to stimulate more normal muscle tone and thereby reduce painful spasms and spasticity. It is also considered beneficial in preventing secondary complications which may arise as a result of prolonged immobility, which can include soft tissue tightness, joint stiffness, and pressure areas. Furthermore it is suggested that regular standing may reduce the risk of osteoporosis and improve psychological well-being. Often the involvement of the person's carer is required to assist with the process of standing. Where this is the case, training is necessary to ensure competence and safety in line with moving and handling legislation. The use of electric standing frames, which mechanically move the person from the sitting to standing position is usually recommended. This not only considerably eases the level of effort required by the person assisting, but in some circumstances can enable the person with MS to stand without personal assistance.

Interventions aimed at teaching others how to safely assist with (or take over) the tasks such as walking, climbing stairs, moving in bed, or transferring.

Interventions aimed at improving level of participations

A wide range of environmental modifications are available which may dramatically improve the mobility and functional independence of people with MS. These can be viewed at the level of the individual as well as at a broader societal level:

- Individual level: includes home setup, ramps, lifts, widening of doorways to enable manoeuvrability, level access showers, bath aids, and environmental control systems.
- Societal level: includes accessibility of buildings and public transport systems, footpaths without kerbs, and pedestrian crossings which allow adequate time to cross the street.

Provision of suitable modifications requires assessment from professionals, such as occupational therapists, who are knowledgeable about the specialist equipment involved.

Mobility aids and equipment

Mobility aids and equipment are often crucial to maximize a person's autonomy and to allow safer and more efficient mobility. A wide range of equipment (sometimes referred to as assistive devices) is available to help achieve this.

Some of this equipment is directly related to *walking*, such as:

• Walking aids, including walking sticks and frames.
• Orthoses such as ankle foot orthoses (AFOs) to assist with foot drop.
• Hand rails or bannisters.

Other equipment relates to broader aspects of *mobility*, such as:

• Bed levers, to enable the person to move more easily in and out of the bed.
• Transfer boards (sliding boards) to assist with bed, toilet, bath, chair, and car transfers.
• Hoists (portable and ceiling).
• Standing frames (either electrically or manually operated).

Other equipment relates to *moving around the wider community setting*, such as:

• Wheelchairs and electric scooters.
• Car mobility: after assessment by an occupational therapist, driving may be safely accomplished with the help of hand controls, low-energy steering wheels, and other aids.

Surveys and qualitative studies highlight that the transition from walking (with whatever difficulty) to the use of a wheelchair is seen by many people with MS as a major life transition. As a consequence, making the decision to use a mobility aid (of whatever type, be it a walking stick or a wheelchair) is often very difficult. Perhaps because of this, there are often conflicting views between the professional and the person with MS at this point about these decisions. It is therefore crucial that the multidisciplinary team introduce the idea of the use of any aids or equipment in a sensitive manner.

There are a range of issues to consider when deciding about which aids and equipment should be provided. These include: the person and their abilities; the phase of MS; current symptoms; the activities that the person wishes to engage in while using the equipment; and the environment in which they will be using it. Having considered all of these issues it is also important to hold discussions about the pros and cons of using the equipment. Potential benefits of using a walking aid can include reduced effort of walking and therefore reduced fatigue, increased stability, and increased safety. Potential benefits of using a wheelchair, for example, can include increased autonomy, reduced fatigue, and reduced spasms and spasticity. Potential disadvantages however are that environmental modifications may be necessary to accommodate the equipment, or that the person's self esteem may be negatively affected. Consideration of this range of issues is essential since failure to consider them can impact markedly on how successfully the individual's needs are met. Furthermore it may have significant cost implications if the equipment does not meet the longer-term needs of the individual. Studies have shown that it is very common for aids and equipment to be assigned to the back of the cupboard, or left on the shelf to accumulate dust, which is clearly wasteful both in economic and personal terms.

While clear and comprehensive professional advice should be given, ultimately the use of the equipment should be left to the decision of the person with MS. The key role of the professional (who is usually the physiotherapist or occupational therapist) is to guide and support the person in making the best choice for themself at that point in time.

Wheelchairs, posture, and seating equipment

Wheelchairs are vital for people with MS who are unable to walk, or who have difficulty with walking. Their use can promote independence, improve function, and enhance quality of life. Current estimates suggest that approximately 25% of people will eventually need to use a wheelchair on a full-time basis. Part-time use, which is often used to enhance autonomy (for example in situations such as when travelling, shopping, or outdoor activities with friends) has been reported in approximately 60% of people.

Functionally, seating and mobility issues cannot be considered separately. Determining the amount and type of support a person needs is a key clinical decision since it directly affects the user's performance within the chair. Inadequate support will not only compromise a person's functional abilities, but it will also promote poor posture, potentially resulting in pain and discomfort. Other long-term consequences of prolonged poor posture include increased incidence of pressure sores, the development of contractures, and cardio-respiratory complications such as decreased respiratory volume.

Key considerations in the selection of mobility and seating equipment

Matching of the individual to the wheelchair and seating system

Some of the key considerations which should be taken into account when considering the individual are their:

- Goals and preferences regarding mobility.
- Physical capabilities and limitations.
- Cognitive abilities, which might for instance impact on their ability to safely manoeuvre powered mobility equipment; and on training requirements.
- Daily activities and lifestyle.
- Resources, such as the social support available and (if a private purchase) finances both in purchasing the system and maintaining it over the longer term.

Anthropometry of the wheelchair and seating system

This deals with aspects related to the dimensions of the wheelchair and seating system, and the person who is sitting in it. Key considerations here are factors such as the size, shape and manoeuvrability of the wheelchair. This includes aspects such as seat depth and width, seat and backrest angle, armrest and back rest height, type and size of wheels and castors.

The physical environments in which the wheelchair will be used

These include:

- The home environment, thinking about issues such as the amount of space required for turning and transfers; the ability to position the chair near items to be reached such as tabletops; access issues such as doorway widths, degree of inclines, floor coverings.

• Access to environments and activities outside of the home, including issues such as transportation, employment environments, and leisure activities.

Appropriate selection of mobility and seating equipment requires a comprehensive assessment, which includes an understanding of the person's physical, cognitive and social situation, as well as knowledge of the previous equipment they have used. Referral to specialist seating and mobility clinics, such as those sited in regional disablement services, is often necessary for those with more complex seating and mobility needs. Typically these services are comprised of teams of physiotherapists and occupational therapists with specialist knowledge in the wide range of equipment available.

Unlike static diseases such as stroke or spinal cord injury, the unpredictable and potentially progressive nature of MS means that the equipment needs of a person with MS will most likely vary over time. This of course makes the selection of equipment even more complicated. Where possible, some attempt should be made to select equipment which is likely to have more long-lived benefit. Providing modular equipment with adjustability in frame and seating parameters for both manual and power wheelchairs increases the long-term flexibility to modify the system as needs change.

Regular reassessments are also necessary to monitor changes in physical, cognitive, and functional status. These enable the clinician to determine whether modifications to existing equipment are needed or whether new equipment is necessary to optimize safety, comfort, function, and continued independence in wheelchair mobility.

Types of wheelchairs and mobility devices

Wheelchairs can be classified as being manual or power driven.

Manual wheelchairs

Based on their purpose and features, manual wheelchairs are further described as standard, performance, or positioning.

Standard wheelchairs refer to basic wheelchairs, which are made of heavier materials and have limited adjustability. They are often used as transport devices in institutional settings. These chairs are not recommended for someone who is a full-time wheelchair user because they do not provide the adjustability that is often needed, and are heavy to self-propel. Their portability however enables them to be used as backup chairs, especially for power wheelchair users who do not have a means of transporting their power chairs in a car or van.

When physical deficits are relatively mild, people may only require a wheelchair intermittently, for example when needing to get about over longer distances or more difficult terrain (such as steeper gradients), or when they are fatigued. In general, provision of a standard wheelchair, with a standard cushion, is sufficient for this purpose, particularly if they will be pushed in the chair by another person.

Performance wheelchairs refer to manual wheelchairs that are made of lighter weight materials and have components that can be adjusted for a more individualized fit. These more specialized wheelchairs are often required as people become more heavily reliant on a wheelchair for their mobility. Some of the available adjustments enable changes to rear wheel positioning for more efficient propulsion, seat-to-back angle for accommodation of the patient's posture, and seat inclination to assist with postural stability. Full-time wheelchair users often need this adjustability to maximize functional mobility.

Self-propulsion in a wheelchair is effortful. This can be a particular problem for many people with MS who suffer from weakness or fatigue. Lightweight wheelchairs can go some way to addressing these difficulties. They are also advantageous for carers, who often find it difficult to lift the chair into car boots or to push them over longer distances on more difficult terrain.

Manual positioning wheelchairs include tilt-in-space and recliner wheelchairs. These chairs are often recommended for people who are dependent for propulsion and repositioning and cannot use a power driven wheelchair.

The tilt-in-space wheelchair is designed to enable a carer to change the person's position in space so that their hips and knees remain at the same angle of approximately 90° when tilted (Fig. 29.2). In doing so the person with MS does not need to be repositioned when moved back to an upright position. The tilt range on these chairs is typically between 0–55°. Typically tilt-in-space chairs are used in people who have significant weakness in their trunk and limbs, and/or those who fatigue easily which means they have difficulty sitting upright all day. The tilted position assists trunk and head control, thereby helping to maintain improved posture and comfort. Importantly it allows the person to rest without moving from their chair. Tilting also enables pressure redistribution from the buttocks to the back, thereby helping to maintain good skin integrity. A disadvantage of tilt-in-space wheelchairs is that they are heavier than other types of manual wheelchairs and are not generally suitable for self-propulsion.

Reclining chairs enable carers to open the seat-to-back angle to assist the person in pressure relief or repositioning (Fig. 29.3).This option can be useful for people who do not have sufficient hip flexion range or who cannot tolerate sitting upright at a fixed hip angle. There are three main drawbacks of the recliner wheelchair:

- The reclined angle promotes a posterior pelvic tilt, which often causes the person to slide forward on the seat. This can cause shearing forces on the buttocks which may damage the soft tissues and cause pressure areas.
- Maintaining the person's seated alignment after the back angle is reclined and brought back upright can be difficult, and repositioning may prove very effortful for the carer.
- The more extended position may increase spasticity or spasms. For example, increased extensor spasticity may occur with backwards thrusting of the head and trunk, or conversely flexor spasms may be triggered by the stretch on tightened hip flexors as the chair is reclined backwards.

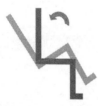

Fig. 29.2 Tilt system: seating angles remain fixed.

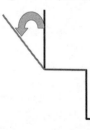

Fig. 29.3 Recliner system: back and seat angles change.

Powered devices

Powered mobility devices, which include folding and non-folding powered wheelchairs and powered scooters, can benefit people with MS by enabling them to conserve energy, decrease fatigue, and participate in activities of daily living. They may be suitable for a wide range of people, although a comprehensive assessment and trial is needed for those with cognitive, perceptual, or visual deficits.

Power chairs can be fitted with seating function options which further enhance the client's mobility, comfort, alignment, and independence. The four commonly used power seat functions are tilt, recline, seat elevator, and elevating legrests. These are important to consider, given the progressive nature of MS.

Some people prefer to use a power scooter over a power wheelchair for aesthetic reasons. Scooters however are only appropriate for people who do not need significant postural support and do not anticipate significant decline in physical function, since they have very basic seat and back cushions that cannot be modified for posture, and cannot accept power seating components such as tilt and recline.

Specialized seating equipment

The aim of specialized seating equipment is to:
• Provide comfort.
• Optimize stability, balance and function.
• Optimize alignment in order to prevent secondary complications such
  as soft tissue and joint contractures, pressure areas, the development
  of scoliosis and respiratory complications.
• Allow equal distribution of load to provide maximal pressure relief.
• Reduce the effort and cost of care.

The need for such equipment is particularly relevant in people whose
motor impairments render them largely inactive, thereby placing them at
a high risk of developing secondary complications. This risk is particularly
great with the presence of severe spasticity and spasms, or marked
weakness, where the body is essentially at the mercy of unopposed
forces. It is now recognized that, in these people, medical and therapy
interventions in isolation are largely ineffective in preventing secondary
complications. Effective management requires a '24-hour postural management approach' to care. Seating is an important component of this
package of postural care, since, for many people, a large proportion of
their day is spent sitting in a chair or wheelchair.

Types of specialist seating equipment

A variety of specialist seating equipment for wheelchairs is available.
Essentially it can be divided into equipment providing support at the seat;
back rest; armrest; footrest and headrest. A brief description of some of
these follows:

Seat support

The seat support is the surface under the buttocks and thighs. Appropriate
seat support is critical in creating good lower-extremity alignment,
pressure relief, and comfort. The support should promote symmetrical
pressure distribution to assist in preventing pressure areas. This requires
that it is of appropriate depth; too short and there will be excessive
pressure under the thighs and a greater risk of lower limb malalignment
(such as windswept legs); too long and it will force the pelvis into
posterior tilt (which will increase the risk of sacral pressure areas) and the
thoracic spine into excessive flexion (which may result in low back pain).
   Improved support can be achieved through the use of specialist
equipment such as:
• Pressure relieving cushions, which can be contoured to provide specific
  support (refer to Chapter 30 on aids and equipment, section on
  pressure relieving cushions).
• Lateral leg supports to maintain the lower limbs in optimal alignment.

Back support

Adequate back support is critical to optimize trunk posture, in particular
to prevent kyphosis or scoliosis and maintain stability. This is important
since trunk posture can impact dramatically on head and upper limb function, respiratory function, and comfort. Specialist equipment, designed to

optimize trunk posture, typically provides external support to help control muscle weakness and trunk asymmetries. Some examples of this equipment include:

- Lateral trunk supports.
- More supportive devices such as the use of matrix or moulded foam carve posture systems. These systems are moulded to individual requirements, and can therefore accommodate fixed structural deformity, and provide a large base of support in order to maximize weight distribution.

To be effective in maintaining good postural alignment, this equipment must not be considered in isolation, but should be viewed together with other seating issues, which include: the angles between the supporting surfaces (seat to back angle, seat to leg angle, leg to foot angle); and position in space (for example by using tilt-in-space systems). By the time that these specialist options are being used, the person's motor impairments are typically so severe that independent function is severely limited. Often the primary aim of seating at this stage is to achieve maximum comfort, pressure relief, stability, and optimal alignment, in order to prevent or arrest the progression of deformity. Functional goals are usually focused on issues such as improving swallowing by optimizing head, neck and trunk alignment; and improving respiratory function by enabling the mechanical work of breathing to be more efficient.

Armrest support

Good arm positioning is important to increase a person's comfort in sitting by having shoulders and arms supported. It can also enhance a person's ability to undertake pressure-relieving strategies such as shifting weight within the chair. Most wheelchairs have adjustable and removable armrests which enable some limited flexibility with height adjustment, and the ability to remove them to ease transfers. More specialist features include: swing away armrests to accommodate transfer style; full-length armrests to assist the person to stand from the wheelchair; or trays to offer increased support.

Footrest support

Approximately 10% of weight is distributed through the feet when seated. Foot contact on the supporting surface is important not only for balance, stability and postural alignment, but also for comfort and pressure relief. Paying attention to foot positioning is therefore an essential part of overall postural management. Impairments such as clonus, spasticity and spasms may result in the feet sliding or spasming off the foot support surface. Soft tissue contractures of muscles surrounding the foot and ankle may mean that the feet cannot rest on the support surface. Adjustable angle footrests and customized footrests are available to help manage these problems.

Headrest support
Control of the head position is particularly challenging, in part because it is dependent upon the alignment and control of other body parts. Headrests help to support and stabilize the head when weakness of the neck muscles and/or fatigue is a major problem. A limited range of different options are available which provide varying levels of support. These include contoured headrests, and those with lateral pads.

Advances in technology mean that a wider range of specialist seating systems is increasingly being made available to help manage postural difficulties, making it difficult for the average clinician to keep abreast of product developments. These specialist systems are generally expensive. These factors combine to make the selection process difficult. Choices should be determined by effective assessment and close discussion with those who will be using the equipment (the person with MS, their carer, and care staff). Working with a knowledgeable team to evaluate equipment options helps to enable the appropriate provision of equipment. While simpler seating systems are generally prescribed by local wheelchair services, complex needs require specialist input from regional centres. These centres have access to a broad range of relevant equipment and personnel, including occupational therapists, physiotherapists, rehabilitation engineers, and wheelchair technicians, whose remit it is to keep abreast of different products on the market.

Chapter 30

Assistive aids and equipment, adaptations, and personal support

Introduction

At some point in time most people with MS will need to use some form of equipment, and/or require some level of personal support, be it on an informal basis from family members, or on a more formal basis from health and social care staff. The variable nature of the symptoms (such as fatigue and spasticity), together with the unpredictable and potentially progressive course of the disease, mean that the type of equipment and level of personal support needed will usually vary over time. Where possible, attempts should be made to select equipment which is likely to have more long-lived benefit. This can be extremely difficult, particularly when dealing with personal support issues.

A detailed and comprehensive assessment of the person's individual needs is essential to ensure appropriate selection of aids and equipment, and recommendations for personal support. Central to this must be a real appreciation of their personal wishes, expectations, and goals. This requires an understanding of their physical, cognitive, emotional and social situation, as well as knowledge of the previous equipment they have used, or personal support they have received.

Given the variable nature of the disease, regular reassessments are necessary to closely monitor changes so that decisions can be made about whether modifications to existing equipment are needed, or whether new equipment or different levels of personal support are necessary. Self-referral review systems offer flexibility to the person with MS so that timely decisions can be made about any changes which are necessary to their care as the changes occur.

Training requirements

The effective use of any piece of equipment requires training of everyone who will use it. This includes the person with MS, their family, and the health and social service staff who are involved in their care. This training should not only include the mechanics of how to use the equipment, but should address issues relating to the underlying cause of the problems, the reason why the equipment is needed, and key principles of care to ensure that a proactive, consistent and 24-hour approach to care is provided to minimize further problems. Along similar lines, there should be training of staff to ensure personal care is provided in the best way possible. For instance, training may be required in the most effective and comfortable way of moving, handling and positioning a person who requires help with this; or in helping to feed, dress, or wash them in a way that is sensitive and appropriate to their needs.

Assistive aids and equipment

Assistive aids and equipment (also referred to as assistive technology devices) refers to any specialist equipment and adaptations, whether off the shelf, modified or customized, which makes performing everyday activities easier. These devices can be mechanical, electronic, manual, or computerized. Very often the right aids can allow people to carry out their daily activities such as cooking, gardening, reading, participating in sports, and continuing to work. For a significant number of people with MS, assistive aids and equipment will be required for many years of their life. The range of aids and equipment available to choose from is enormous. Some examples include:

- Devices to aid in activities of daily living, such as button hooks for dressing, and rocker knives for cutting food.
- Kitchen equipment, such as perching stools, kettle pourers, mobile trays, or pot and pan stabilizers.
- Bathroom or toilet equipment, such as shower chairs, bath seats, bath boards and raised toilet seats.
- Intercom or environmental control systems.
- Equipment related to work, such as special grips for pens and pencils, specialist computer equipment such as adaptive keyboard and mouse equipment, as well as assistive hardware and software.

Effective use of equipment can bring enormous benefits to the person with MS, and to their carer. For instance they may:

- Enhance independence.
- Be a useful energy conservation strategy for managing fatigue.
- Reduce burden and minimize stress on carers.
- Enable people to remain in their homes for longer.
- Improve quality of life.

Most technical aids and equipment are prescribed by occupational therapists and provided through health or social services. Occupational therapists are qualified to undertake assessment of individual need based on task performance, to discuss with the person what their individuals needs are, and to provide specialist instructions and recommendations about the use of equipment. Aids focusing on assisting mobility are typically prescribed by physiotherapists, and aids for assisting communication are prescribed by speech and language therapists. At other times people with MS purchase equipment privately themselves, often with no advice other than that of the sales person.

Effective prescription of assistive aids and equipment is essential since it makes up a substantial portion of the direct cost of MS. Probably the most important basis for evaluating an assistive device is whether it satisfies the needs of the person for whom it is prescribed, as demonstrated by the fact that they use it. Unfortunately research shows that resources are often wasted as people are provided with equipment (or select and purchase it themselves) but then recognize after using it that it does not meet their needs and so abandon its use, This 'abandonment', which is estimated to occur in approximately one third of cases, typically occurs immediately or within the first year following obtainment of the equipment, and has found to be influenced by a number of factors (Table 30.1).

This clearly has significant implications, both with respect to the wasted resources which might be better spent elsewhere but perhaps more importantly to the potential lost benefits to the person whose needs are not being met. It cannot be overemphasized how important it is for the person with MS to be actively involved in the decision-making process since it is they that best know their lifestyle and whether they will incorporate use of any equipment within it. Table 30.2 outlines some key questions that should be asked and answered prior to prescribing or purchasing aids and equipment. Consideration of these issues may go some way to help ensure that equipment is prescribed which will be used by, and be useful to, those affected by MS.

Table 30.1 Factors which influence abandonment of assistive aids and equipment

- Lack of consideration of user opinion in selection of the equipment.
- Poor equipment performance.
- Change in the needs of the user.
- Lack of information and training.
- Inappropriate prescription of equipment.
- Non-acceptance of the equipment (as it may be seen as a symbol of being ill, 'giving in to the disease', or losing independence).
- Equipment which is unattractive.

Table 30.2 Key questions to ask and answer before prescribing or purchasing aids and equipment:

Portability and mobility:
- Can the equipment be taken apart, reassembled, and lifted by the person with MS or a family member (e.g. putting a wheelchair or scooter in a car)?
- Does the equipment easily fit into the person's home or anywhere else they plan on using it (e.g. workplace, shops, cars, and public transportation)?
- Do they have adequate space to store the equipment?
- Is the equipment appropriate for how they want to use it (e.g. type of wheelchair)?

Appearance and comfort:
- Will the person feel comfortable using the aid in public?
- Is it comfortable for them to wear?
- Can it be adjusted to fit the person's height, weight, shape, and personal preferences?
- Does the person feel secure and safe while using the equipment?

Changing needs:
- Will the equipment meet the person's needs (or can it be modified to meet their needs) if their condition changes?

Quality and ease of use:
- Will the equipment help the person to accomplish activities they want to do?
- Is there anyone they can talk to who uses the device?
- Can they get training to use the device?
- Can they try out several devices before making a selection?
- Does the equipment have a warranty? And what is the returns policy (if privately purchased)?
- Does the device require batteries? If so, how often do the batteries need to be replaced and/or recharged?
- What is the sales person's experience and training (if equipment is being privately purchased)?
- Can the person afford to maintain the device (if privately purchased)?
- Will they be able to receive technical support if they have difficulty with the device?

After Dent E, and Holberg C. Purchasing assistive technology? Ask the right questions! *MS Care* Autumn 2005; 117–20. Available at: *http://www.mscare.com*.

Equipment for postural control and pressure care

People who are more severely affected by MS can often find it difficult to change their body posture or position independently, and as a result they may sit in static, habitual, and often asymmetrical postures. This places them at risk of developing contractures, deformities or pressure areas, which in turn can have profoundly negative consequences on their comfort, functioning, and quality of life. Twenty four-hour postural management is essential to try to prevent this from happening. The aim of this approach is to optimize postural alignment in all of the different positions assumed by the person, and with all of the supportive equipment used by them, throughout the 24-hour period (for instance when sitting in a wheelchair or chair, when standing, and when lying in bed).

Twenty four-hour management requires considerable and sustained commitment from all those caring for the person with MS (both family members and health and social service staff). In addition, specialist aids and equipment are often necessary to enable postural management to be undertaken effectively over the entire period. Described below are some potentially useful aids and equipment which can enhance postural management and positioining, and provide pressure relief. Decisions about aids and equipment should be based on an overall assessment of the person, which incorporates not simply their neuro-musculo-skeletal status, but also other important factors such as their lifestyle, and acceptability of the equipment to them and their family. Cost should also be considered.

Unfortunately, there currently remains a lack of clarity as to whether health or social services are responsible for providing some of this equipment. This can often result in considerable confusion and distress for the person with MS who is typically severely disabled, and who is desperate to maintain their physical status as best as possible in the face of deteriorating neurological status, which is notoriously difficult to manage.

Wedges and t-rolls

The use of equipment such as wedges, t-rolls, or pillows is typically used in people with asymmetry which results from spasticity and spasms, or contractures. By promoting more equal loading of tissues, and improving the alignment of body segments, this equipment can be useful both in preventing and arresting contractures and pressure sores, and improving comfort. Clinically it is observed that the severity of spasms and spasticity is often reduced (or made more manageable), by enabling the limbs to rest into the support it offers. This equipment, which is usually prescribed by a physiotherapist, is relatively inexpensive, and can be used both within the home and hospital setting.

Beds, mattresses, and overlays for pressure relief

A wide range of pressure-relieving beds, mattresses, and overlays are used, both within community and hospital settings. The aim of this equipment is to prevent pressure areas in people who are at high risk of developing them. These include people who have reduced mobility, or are immobile; sensory impairment; spasticity and/or spasms; or are incontinent. This type of equipment is usually categorized according to whether it is a 'low tech' or 'high tech' device, as follows:

- Low tech devices are those that provide a conforming support surface that distributes the body weight over a large area. These include:
  - Foam alternatives to standard mattresses, such as high specification foam or cubed foam.
  - Gel filled, fluid filled or air filled mattresses/overlays
- High tech devices are dynamic systems that use an alternating support surface, typically where inflatable cells alternately inflate and deflate. These include:
  - Alternating pressure mattresses/overlays.
  - Air fluidized beds/mattresses/overlays.
  - Low air loss beds/mattresses/overlays.
  - Electric profiling beds, turning beds or frames.

While the evidence from randomized controlled trials shows that each of these devices reduces the incidence of pressure areas, a recent systematic review shows that there is insufficient evidence to support the use of one type over another[1]. The NICE guidelines on the use of pressure relieving devices for the prevention of pressure ulcers[2] recommends that, at a minimum, all individuals who are assessed as being vulnerable to pressure areas should use a high specification (low tech) foam mattress with pressure relieving properties. While acknowledging the lack of research evidence to support the use of high tech pressure relieving mattresses over low tech mattresses, they do however recommend that consideration should be given to the use of alternating pressure or other high tech pressure relieving systems.

Sleeping systems

Sleeping systems provide adjustable support which is customized to the individual. They are relatively expensive and are not commonly provided by health or social services. These systems are typically used by people who are unable (or virtually unable) to move, and who require significant postural support and pressure relief when lying in bed. Their use is designed to optimize body symmetry, thereby preventing (or arresting) musculoskeletal problems such as contractures, pain, and pressure sores. They are also reported to reduce tone abnormalities. By improving the quality and comfort of the person's sleep, family members and carers are also less frequently disturbed since the person is able to remain in a supported and comfortable position for longer periods of time. A number of systems are currently available, which include the Symmetrisleep system and the Dreama system.

---

1 Cullum M, McInnes E, Bell-Syer SEM, *et al.* Support surfaces for pressure ulcer prevention. *The Cochrane Database of Systematic Reviews* 2006, Issue 1.
2 *The NICE guidelines on the use of pressure relieving devices (beds, mattresses and overlays) for the prevention of pressure ulcers in primary and secondary care, Clinical Guideline 7, October 2003.* Available at: www.nice.org.uk

Wheelchairs and specialist seating equipment

This has been discussed in some detail in Chapter 29 on Mobility issues.

Specialist pressure relieving cushions for sitting

A wide range of specialist seating cushions are available. Research suggests that no single cushion is optimal in relieving pressure, or providing optimal postural management, for all patients. As with all other aids and equipment, an assessment of the person's specific needs is required. There are a number of different features which should be considered when deciding which cushion is most appropriate, some of which include:

- Conformity: some cushions are made of substances that move and conform to the shape of the body, e.g. air, water, gel. This type of cushion is ideal for distributing pressure as it forms a large surface over which areas of high pressure can be dispersed. However, cushions that conform easily have disadvantages in that pressure cannot be relieved by leaning forwards or to one side, since the cushion will move as the body moves. Similarly, they do not provide help when transferring since if the person needs to push down on the cushion to gain some leverage, the contents of the cushion will move as soon as the body weight is lifted.
- Shear forces: some cushions are designed to reduce shear forces as much as possible. For instance cushions that have an individual balloon or egg-box shaped surface, or foam cushions which have a surface of individual foam cubes, are able to move with the body so that the pull on the outer layer of skin is decreased. Cushions which are ramped backwards decrease the likelihood of the person sliding forwards in the chair, thereby reducing shearing forces on the tissues.
- Stability: when the person has poor postural control it can be difficult for them to maintain sitting balance. When this is the case cushions that easily conform to the body and its movements often do not provide adequate stability for the person and they can sometimes feel unsafe. When this is the case a more stable cushion, that has good pressure relieving properties, is often preferable.
- Weight: and hence portability of the cushion, is important to consider if the person needs to frequently lift it on and off the wheelchair, or in and out of the car. Some cushion materials, such as gel or water, are heavy and, even with handles on the covers, are not easy to lift. This can be particularly important for someone who experiences muscle weakness or fatigue.

Home adaptations

Home adaptations are permanent alterations to a home, often involving some building work. These adaptations typically aim to promote safety in the home and to enable the person to live there more independently.

Some examples of home adaptations include:
- Accessible toilets, showers and baths
- Widened doors
- Lowered surfaces and sockets
- Fitted handrails
- Ramps
- Hoists
- Lifts.

Usually an occupational therapist makes an assessment as to which adaptations are most appropriate for the person. Based on this assessment, the adaptations may be undertaken, either by social services, or on a private basis.

Personal care

Unpaid care giving from informal support networks, such as family members and friends, has now been recognized as providing a major proportion of the care that is given to people with MS. It is probably the critical factor which enables people to remain living in their own homes. In trying to meet the physical, emotional and social needs of the person with MS, family members and friends often carry a considerable burden of physical work and emotional strain. This can be extremely stressful and exhausting, and at times overwhelming, particularly when help may be needed constantly and over a long time. The changing role, restriction on time and freedom, and potential changes in employment status can also result in a change in the relationship between the person with MS and the family member. It is important that practical help is provided from relevant health and social care services, where it is required, and when the person with MS and their family wish it. Occasionally, family members prefer to be the sole providers of care, and when this is the case this should be respected. More commonly, however, people are desperate to receive more help.

The majority of care packages wherein people are cared for within their home setting are provided by social services. District nursing may also be involved if there is an identifiable nursing need, as will input from other health professionals. Care packages are often led by care team managers whose role is to coordinate the often large number of health and social care personnel who may be required. These packages, which are tailored according to individual need, may include assistance with any combination of the following:

- Personal care such as washing, dressing and feeding.
- Mobility functions such as transferring in and out of bed.
- Domestic tasks such as home help with cleaning.
- Services such as meals on wheels.
- Respite care packages, such as day care centres.

Meeting carers' needs is as important as meeting the needs of the person with MS. Research has demonstrated that 'care givers' with adequate levels of social support are less vulnerable to physical and psychiatric morbidity. Maintaining carers' physical and emotional health is clearly important if people with MS are to live in their own homes for as long as they would like.

Part 5

Evaluation of services

Chapter 31

Evaluation of services

Introduction

The breadth and diversity of services which often needs to be accessed by people with MS throughout the course of their disease is enormous. Even at a single point in time, care delivery may span a number of different organizations and specialities. Any attempt to evaluate the overall pathway of care experienced by a person is therefore fraught with difficulties, and so a pragmatic approach to the evaluation of service delivery is required. One relatively straightforward approach is to evaluate the care provided by discrete services. This might include multidisciplinary services such as diagnostic clinics, inpatient rehabilitation units, respite care services, or uni-disciplinary services. Typically these evaluations will focus on three key aspects of the service, namely its:

- Structures, such as numbers and grading of staff.
- Processes, such as admission and discharge procedures.
- Outcomes, such as patient satisfaction with the service, or clinical outcomes such as level of functional ability or discharge destination.

While valuable information will be gained from these evaluations, a disadvantage of this approach is that an overview of the overall patient journey doesn't occur.

Another useful approach is to evaluate the effectiveness of care in terms of its ability to deal with specific problems faced by the patient. This might include, for instance, the management of acute relapses, or the prevention and management of pressure sores. Because this approach usually involves the evaluation of care which is provided both within and across different services, these evaluations can tap into key aspects of service delivery such as whether mechanisms are in place to facilitate effective transfer between different services and settings; and whether such mechanisms are utilized in a timely and appropriate manner.

Issues pertaining to the evaluation of treatment effectiveness as determined by research studies has been previously discussed (refer to Chapter 10). This chapter focuses, in rather broad terms, on the evaluation of service delivery in routine clinical practice, which is most commonly undertaken through the use of mechanisms such as clinical audit and integrated care pathways.

Clinical audit

Clinical audit is a quality improvement process that seeks to improve patient care and outcomes through systematic evaluation of care against explicit criteria and the implementation of change. All aspects of service delivery (structures, processes, and outcomes of care) can be evaluated using clinical audit.

In brief, a series of steps are undertaken which involves identification of cases, collection of information (typically from patient records) and analysis of data. Where indicated, changes are then implemented at an individual, team or service level and further monitoring is used to confirm improvement in healthcare delivery (Fig. 31.1). Unfortunately in practise the audit process can be hindered by a number of problems. For instance the standard of note keeping usually varies widely, as do the methods of recording information. Outcomes are often not routinely recorded on all patients, nor are they recorded in a standard way. Furthermore, it is common for each profession to write and store their own clinical records, with relatively little sharing of information. These factors all combine to make it difficult to attain the type of information necessary to undertake an audit satisfactorily.

In order to facilitate effective audit, these difficulties can be minimized in the following ways:

- Using structured sets of standardized documentation, such as assessment forms, protocols of care, goal setting, and discharge summaries.
- Agreeing on the areas of outcome to be routinely measured, the standardized methods for undertaking and recording these measures, and the intervals at which the outcomes should be measured.
- Using standardized methods for recording key process issues for the person admitted to the service, such as the use of integrated care pathways.
- Providing leadership in clinical audit.
- Providing ownership of the process by all members of staff.
- Maintaining registers, or databases of persons admitted to a service.
- Using standardized audit packages, where these exist, to enhance comparability between audits and between services.

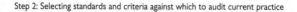

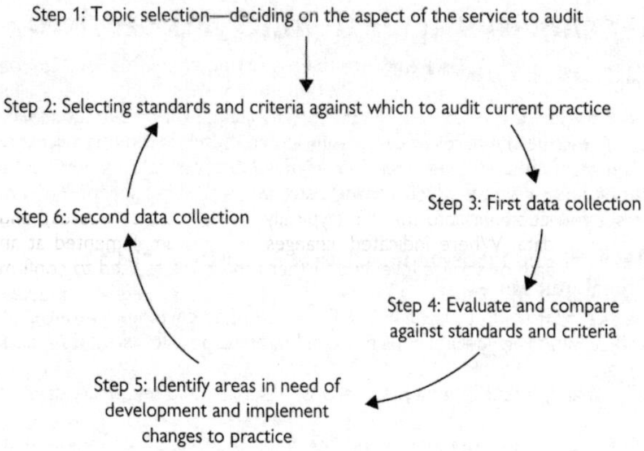

Step 1: Topic selection—deciding on the aspect of the service to audit

Step 2: Selecting standards and criteria against which to audit current practice

Step 3: First data collection

Step 6: Second data collection

Step 4: Evaluate and compare against standards and criteria

Step 5: Identify areas in need of development and implement changes to practice

Fig. 31.1 The audit cycle.

Benchmarks against which MS services can be evaluated

There are a number of key documents, which can be freely accessed, which describe standards of care, against which services can be evaluated. In the main, they provide clear and relatively detailed information about specific audit criteria, which can be used for evaluation purposes. They are summarized below:

The National Institute for Clinical Excellence (NICE) clinical guidelines

The National Institute for Clinical Excellence has developed a range of national clinical guidelines which are relevant to people with MS. These include:

- The management of multiple sclerosis in primary and secondary care (2003).[1]
- The use of pressure relieving devices (beds, mattresses and overlays) for the prevention of pressure ulcers in primary and secondary care (2003).[2]
- Pressure ulcers: the management of pressure ulcers in primary and secondary care (2005).[3]

In order to assist with their implementation into clinical practice, each of these guidelines clearly details the key audit criteria and audit objectives which are associated with the specific evidence based recommendations made.

The 'Management of MS in primary and secondary care' (2003) is a key document against which all services delivering care to people with MS should evaluate their service delivery. This document identifies 6 key priorities for implementation and details suggested measures (criterion: data items needed) for auditing services within the National Health Service. These 6 key priorities are summarized in Table 31.1.

The National Service Framework for long-term conditions

Alongside the national guidelines, the National Service Framework (NSF) for long-term conditions[4] is a major drive for the evaluation of MS services. The NSF sets out 11 quality requirements to improve the way health and social care services support people with long-term neurological conditions to live as independently as possible. This framework emphasizes the need for the development of a more integrated approach to delivering services by increased working between health and social care services and local agencies involved in supporting people to live independently,

1 *Multiple Sclerosis: management of multiple sclerosis in primary and secondary care.* Clinical Guidelines 8, National Institute for Clinical Excellence, November 2003. Available at: www.nice.org.uk
2 *The use of pressure relieving devices (beds, mattresses and overlays) for the prevention of pressure ulcers in primary and secondary care.* Clinical Guideline 7, National Institute for Clinical Excellence October 2003. Available at: www.nice.org.uk
3 *Pressure ulcers: the management of pressure ulcers in primary and secondary care.* Clinical Guideline 29, National Institute for Clinical Excellence, September 1995.
4 *The National Service Framework for long-term conditions.* Department of Health, March 2005.

such as providers of transport, housing, employment, education, benefits, and pensions.

The 11 quality requirements of the NSF (Table 31.2) are the key areas against which services need to develop and be evaluated.

Table 31.1 NICE clinical guidelines for the management of MS: the six key priorities for intervention

Key priority for implementation

1. Specialized services
Specialist neurological and neurological rehabilitation services should be available to every person with MS, when they need them.

2. Rapid diagnosis
An individual who is suspected of having MS should be referred to a specialist neurology service, and seen rapidly within an audited time. The individual should be seen again after all investigations necessary to confirm or refute the diagnosis have been completed.

3. Seamless service
Every health commissioning organization should ensure that all organizations in a local health area agree and publish protocols for sharing and transferring responsibility for and information about people with MS, so as to make the service seamless from the individual's perspective.

4. A responsive service
All services and service personnel within the healthcare sector should recognize—and respond to—the varying and unique needs and expectations of the person with MS. The person with MS should be involved actively in all decisions and actions.

5. Sensitive but thorough problem assessment
Health service professionals in regular contact with people with MS should consider in a systematic way whether the person has a 'hidden' problem contributing to their clinical situation, such as fatigue, depression, cognitive impairment, impaired sexual function, or reduced bladder control.

6. Self-referral after discharge
Every person with MS who has been seen by a specialist neurological or neurological rehabilitation service should be informed about how to make contact with the service when he or she is no longer under regular treatment or review. The individual should be given guidance on when such contact is appropriate.

The British Society for Rehabilitation Medicine's standards for specialist inpatient and community rehabilitation services in the United Kingdom

The British Society of Rehabilitation Medicine has developed clinical standards to allow inpatient rehabilitation services to be evaluated against detailed audit criteria[1]. The following 10 key areas are covered in these standards: service provision, the rehabilitation team, referral and assessment, start of rehabilitation, assessment and programme planning, coordination of the rehabilitation process, discharge, follow-up, staff development/audit and training, and liaison with other healthcare services and agencies. The explicit criteria against which services should be evaluated are freely available from the British Society of Rehabilitation Medicine website, accessible at: http://www.bsrm.co.uk/ClinicalGuidance/ClinicalGuidance.htm.

The MS Society of Great Britain and Northern Ireland's 'Measuring Success Scheme'

The MS Society of Great Britain and Northern Ireland has developed an audit toolkit which is aimed at supporting professionals who wish to develop and evaluate their services. The toolkit focuses the user on appraising how their current (and potential) service provision meets the recommendations made in the NICE clinical guidelines for the management of MS. Importantly it facilitates them to develop action plans to address the issues raised. Table 31.3 provides an example of the audit criteria which are detailed in the toolkit for one of the six key priorities listed in the MS Guidelines.

The 'Measuring Success Scheme' encourages evaluation by both professionals and users of the service. It provides an incentive by awarding those services which demonstrate good practice in the field of MS with the 'Measuring Success Award'.

1 Turner-Stokes L, *et al. Clinical standards for inpatient specialist rehabilitation services in the UK.* Clinical Rehabilitation 2000; **14**: 468–80.

Table 31.2 The eleven quality requirements of the National Service Framework for long-term conditions

Quality requirement

1. A person-centred service.
2. Early recognition, prompt diagnosis and treatment.
3. Emergency and acute management.
4. Early and specialist rehabilitation.
5. Community rehabilitation and support.
6. Vocational rehabilitation.
7. Providing equipment and accommodation.
8. Providing personal care and support.
9. Palliative care.
10. Supporting family and carers.
11. Caring for people with neurological conditions in hospital or other health and social care settings.

Recommendations on Rehabilitation Services for Persons with Multiple Sclerosis in Europe

Two important European forum (RIMS—Rehabilitation in Multiple Sclerosis; and European MS Platform) collaborated to develop these recommendations for MS rehabilitation in Europe[1]. The recommendations, which are fairly broad-based are essentially structured around the key interventions provided by the rehabilitation team and individual disciplines within the team.

---

1 *Recommendations on rehabilitation services for persons with multiple sclerosis in Europe.* Associazione Italiana Sclerosi Multipla, Genoa, Italy, 2002.

Table 31.3 An example of audit criteria from the MS Society's 'Measuring Success' audit toolkit

Key Priority 6

Every person with MS who has been seen by a specialist neurological or neuro-logical rehabilitation service should be informed about how to make contact with the service when he or she is no longer under regular treatment or review. The individual should be given guidance on when such contact is appropriate.

Recommendation 1.2.6.1

When any 'episode of care' (medical or rehabilitation treatment programme) ends (that is, when no further benefit is anticipated), the healthcare team should:

- Ensure that any necessary long-term support needs are met.
- Ensure that the person with MS knows who to contact and how to contact them, in the event that the person with MS experiences a change in their situation.
- Discuss with the person with MS whether they want a regular review of their situation and, if so, agree on a suitable and reasonable interval and method of review (for example, by phone, or post, or as an outpatient).

Audit criteria	Met	Partially met	Not met
The presence or not of a formal procedure for responding to self-referral by someone with MS in the: • Neurology service • Neuro-rehabilitation service.			

Local implementation

- Agree protocol for identifying the specific point of contact for access to local MS services and mechanism for informing people with MS.
- Agree a protocol for instigating regular reviews with a person with MS and how this should be done.
- Establish whether a specialist MS nurse or therapist is available locally and if so, how they are contacted.
- Identify who is responsible for providing and keeping up to date self-help booklets that reflect the priorities of people with MS.
- Compile a list of all relevant local and national organizations involved with MS and ensure that it is kept up to date.
- Compile a list of locally relevant information resources and ensure that this is kept up to date.
- Define responsibility for enabling people with MS to access self-help skills and knowledge.
- Agree an integrated approach to rehabilitation, vocational and leisure services, including defining referral criteria for relevant services and methods for exchanging relevant information.

Reproduced with permission from the *Measuring Success Audit Toolkit*, Multiple Sclerosis Society of Great Britain and Northern Ireland. Accessible at *http://www.mssociety.org.uk*

Integrated care pathways (ICPs)

ICPs are structured multidisciplinary care plans which detail essential steps in the care of patients with a specific clinical problem. They consist of a document which maps the anticipated course of a patient's passage through the health system for a given episode of care, as well as when departures from the expected pathway occur (variances). In doing so they are able to facilitate effective clinical audit by identifying *what* should happen, *when* it should happen, by *whom*, and *why* it may not have happened (variance).

There are a number of benefits to using ICPs, some of which include:
- The provision of consistent and structured information about process.
- The ability to clearly identifiy 'gaps' and duplication in care.
- Increased consistency of care and reduction of risk.
- Improved communication.
- Facilitates proactive discharge planning.
- It is a ready made tool for auditing process and outcome.
- Provides a structure for introducing clinical guidelines.

These benefits do, however, come at a cost. To be effective, commitment is required from all team members, as is regular education to ensure consistency in completion of the forms. This can be difficult, particularly if staff turnover is high. Implementation has proven to be effective within defined settings, such as inpatient rehabilitation units (refer to Tables 31.4 and 31.5 for an example of this). Reports from clinical practice suggest, however, that their use is more problematic in following patients as they are transferred between different settings, for instance from the acute hospital setting to the rehabilitation unit and then on to the community. In the main this is due to practical issues such as the forms being lost, or not fully completed.

Some tips for effective implementation include:
- Ensuring the ICP is patient-centred.
- Ensuring clear, dynamic leadership is in place.
- Supporting implementation with a rolling programme of education.
- Having a key-worker system in place, so that a key person takes responsibility for ensuring the form is completed.
- Using the data, so that staff can understand the benefits to patient care.
- Ensuring the ICP is 'integrated' with existing quality improvement processes.

Table 31.4 An example of a section of an ICP, illustrating how detailed process issues can be documented in a standardized manner to facilitate audit of routine practice

Week 1: Assessment	(Please tick)	Date	Name	Variance code
Medical clerking within 24 hours?	☐ Yes ☐ No			
Patient's joint assessment form completed?	☐ Yes ☐ No			
Joint assessment by team and action plan agreed with patient?	☐ Yes ☐ No			
Joint assessment within 24 hours?	☐ Yes ☐ No			
Key worker present at joint assessment?	☐ Yes ☐ No			
All team members present at joint assessment?	☐ Yes ☐ No			
Carer present at joint assessment?	☐ Yes ☐ No ☐ N/A			
Medical notes/films/reports received?	☐ Yes ☐ No ☐ N/A			
Nursing notes received? *(Separate tick boxes are allocated for identifying whether notes for all other team members have been received)*	☐ Yes ☐ No ☐ N/A			
Transfer method agreed?	☐ Yes ☐ No ☐ N/A			
Wheelchair seating/posture assessment commenced?	☐ Yes ☐ No ☐ N/A			

Table 31.5 A small selection of some of the variance codes detailed for this ICP

Variance codes Patient/Condition	Code	Internal System	Code
Patient medically deteriorated	05	Date or time of treatment changed	210
Patient cognitive difficulties	10	Planned meeting cancelled	220
Patient fatigue	20	Goal timing inappropriate	240
Neurological deterioration	30	(Named discipline) not available	260–276
Patient/Carer		Reduced staffing (named discipline)	311–315
Patient not available but on unit	110	Equipment not available	320
Patient not on unit	131	**External system**	
Patient declines treatment	140	Home care not yet available	410
Patient disagrees with goals	150	Follow-up therapy not available	470
Carers unavailable	180	Funding difficulties	480

Integrated Care Pathway, version 2.0 from the National Hospital of Neurology and Neurosurgery Rehabilitation Unit, Queen Square, London. Reproduced with permission.

Seeking the views of service users

The perceptions of service users are an extremely important and useful way of planning and evaluating health and social care services. Importantly they can keep services focused on providing patient centred services. Patients and carers opinions can be gathered in a range of different ways, some of which include:

- Informal conversations.
- Focus groups and forums involving patients.
- Surveys, which may include patient satisfaction questionnaires.
- Interviews of service users.
- Involvement of people affected by MS in research projects aimed at evaluating services.

Table 31.6 provides an example of the types of questions that surveys can use to explore the views of people with MS about their experiences of health services. These questions are reproduced from a survey undertaken by the Royal College of Physicians and the MS Trust, which asks specific questions relating to the implementation of the key recommendations made in the 2003 NICE guidelines. Using a 360° approach, separate questionnaires were sent to people with MS, and to healthcare and primary care trusts across six strategic health authorities in England. The information generated by surveys of this nature, which can be undertaken at either a local or national level, can provide a useful picture of the quality of health care services provided for people with MS.

Table 31.6 A sample of questions asked in a survey seeking the views of people with MS about their experiences of health services

Section: Diagnosis in the last 12 months

If you were diagnosed in the last 12 months, please complete this section.

6. Were you given any of the following information upon your diagnosis?

YES	NO	
☐	☐	Information booklet about MS
☐	☐	Contact details of an MS specialist nurse
☐	☐	Information on how to see a specialist if you develop a problem
☐	☐	Guidance regarding MS support groups
☐	☐	Information regarding education programmes
☐	☐	Other (please specify)

7. If you were referred with suspected MS in the last year, were you seen by a specialist neurologist within 6 weeks?

☐ YES ☐ NO

8. Were all tests completed within 6 weeks of first consultation?

☐ YES ☐ NO

9. How long did it take from seeing your GP to getting the results of all the tests?

☐ 1–6 weeks ☐ 7–10 weeks ☐ 10–15 weeks ☐ 16 weeks or more

10. If there were any delays, were they explained to you?

☐ YES ☐ NO

If you would like to make any further comment about your diagnosis procedure please feel free to do so.

_____

_____

Survey questions taken from a 360° survey undertaken by the Royal College of Physicians and the MS Trust in 2006. Reproduced with permission.

Core competencies of staff

Key competencies for specialist MS nurses[1] and therapists[2] have been developed, which provide a structure against which it is possible to describe (and perhaps even evaluate) the knowledge, skills and competence of professionals specializing in the field of MS. The specialist MS nurses make use of a competency framework to achieve this. This framework describes the range of work activities that need to be carried out to achieve the objectives of the organisation (or occupational sector), together with the quality standards to which these activities need to be performed. In doing so it aims to facilitate nurses in maping their own development within their clinical role, thereby helping them to evaluate their effectiveness within that role. Table 31.7 provides a brief outline of some of the key competencies which have been described for specialist MS nurses and therapists.

1 *Competencies for MS Specialist Nurses*, MS Trust, MS Specialist Nurse Association and Royal College of Nursing, July 2003. Available from *http://www.mstrust.org.uk*
2 *Therapists in MS: delivering the long-term solutions*, MS Trust March 2006. Available from *http://www.mstrust.org.uk*

Table 31.7 Key competencies for specialist MS nurses and therapists

Specialist nursing competencies

- In depth knowledge of MS across the disease spectrum.
- Advanced clinical assessment and management skills.
- Expertise in communication and coordination skills to ensure service is responsive to changing need; to allow self-management, and access to services when required.
- Effective relationship and advocacy skills which facilitate a trusting relationship between the person with MS, and the development of effective services.
- Effective in prioritizing work load and resources, and in developing effective administration services to support service provision.
- Effective in working in different health and social environments, and in establishing working relationships that promote partnership between health, social, voluntary, and independent sectors.
- Lead the development of policies affecting the care of people with MS, reflecting local and national priorities.
- Effective in teaching and sharing knowledge, across a range of different settings and at a range of levels.
- Undertake audit and research, and use the results of research effectively.

Specialist therapy competencies

- In depth knowledge of MS across the disease spectrum.
- High level therapy skills and advanced clinical reasoning.
- Extensive clinical experience of treating different types of MS.
- Highly effective communication skills.
- Networking skills and knowledge of national, regional, and local facilities/staff.
- A passion for MS management.
- Focused approach.
- Foresight, gained through knowledge and experience about what may happen.

Summarized from: *Competencies for MS Specialist Nurses*, July 2003; and *Therapists in MS: delivering the long-term solutions*, March 2006.

Part 6

Useful resources

Useful resources

Introduction

An enormous amount of information is available to people living with MS and to professionals involved in their management. Unfortunately while this is generally helpful, at times it can be overwhelming, confusing, and sometimes contradictory. It is therefore important to encourage all those affected by MS to view the available information in a critical light. The following provides a list of some valuable sources of balanced, reliable and up-to-date information on issues related to MS.

Support from charitable bodies

There are a number of voluntary organizations who provide valuable advice and information to support people with MS, their families and friends, and all health professionals who work with them. Importantly the information is presented in patient friendly terms, in a variety of formats.

The core services typically provided by these organizations include:

- Telephone help-lines.
- Electronic chatrooms. These can include different forums such as advice help-lines, question and answer sessions hosted by experts, and discussion groups where people can share experiences, advice and information.
- Publications on all aspects related to MS and living with the condition. These are typically available in a variety of different formats including books, pamphlets, reports and multimedia. They cover a wide diversity of areas such as diagnosis; diet and nutrition; sex, intimacy and relationships; benefits; respite, and long-term care.
- Websites where the majority of publications can be freely downloaded.
- Regular updates about the latest medical developments, including clinical trials, via member newsletters and the website.
- Information about local and regional branches, which includes information about local support services and training days.
- Information about relevant international, national and local conferences, or courses.

The National MS Society of Great Britain and Northern Ireland *http://www.mssociety.org.uk*

This is the website for the National MS Society of Great Britain and Northern Ireland. It provides access to all of the core services described above. Some particularly useful documents include:

- *MS Essentials*, a series of evidence based publications on a wide range of topics.
- Links to key guidance documents including *The National Clinical Guidelines for MS Management: The Physiotherapy Guidance Document* related to these guidelines; *The National Service Framework for long-term conditions*.
- Monthly research bulletins which summarize studies recently published in reputable journals.

The MS Trust
http://www.mstrust.org.uk

The MS Trust is an independent UK charity. As well as providing many of the core services described above, it has a number of documents which are useful in developing MS specific services. These documents include:

- *Therapists in MS—delivering the long-term solutions*: which highlights the specialist role played by therapists and the benefits this can bring to patient care.

- *Competencies for MS specialist nurses*: which provides guidance on the competencies required by MS nurses and helps the identification of training and educational needs.
- *Specialist Nursing in MS—the way forward*: which gives detailed guidance on the development of MS nurse specialist posts, identifies the development requirements of post-holders, considers different models of care, and suggests standards of clinical operation.
- MS information updates, which provide a quarterly listing of recent papers published in the field of MS.

The National MS Society
http://www.nationalmssociety.org

This is the website of the National MS Society of America. Some particularly useful documents include:

- 'Clinical Bulletins', a series of publications providing guidance for professionals about a broad range of areas.
- Expert opinion papers, providing consensus statements about treatment recommendations including disease management and rehabilitation.
- Links to the American Academy of Neurology guidelines on clinical practice in relation to a wide range of treatment areas including: utility of MRI in suspected MS; use of disease modifying therapies, and the use of corticosteroids.

Useful websites for the multidisciplinary team

The Consortium of MS Centres (CMSC)
http://www.mscare.org

CMSC is a multidisciplinary organization providing a team approach to MS care and a network for all health care professionals and others specializing in the care of people with MS. Within this site are a range of evidence-based guidelines for professionals, which have been developed by the Multiple Sclerosis Council for clinical practice guidelines. These include guidelines on:

- Fatigue management
- Bladder management
- Spasticity management.

The *International Journal of MS Care*, which is published on a quarterly basis, can also be freely accessed via this website. This journal contains articles on a wide range of topics of interest to those involved in the health and social care of people with MS.

International organization of MS Nurses (IOMSN)
http://www.iomsn.org/

This is the website for the international organization of MS nurses. It focuses on the needs and goals of professional nurses who care for people with MS. Some particularly useful aspects include:

- Monographs about important nursing issues including case management and best nursing practice.
- Roundtable discussion forums about key nursing issues, such as managing patient expectations.

Other useful sources of information

The Cochrane Library and Controlled Trials Register

http:www.cochrane.org

The Cochrane Collaboration is an international, independent organisation, whose primary aim is to make up-to-date, accurate information about the effects of healthcare readily available worldwide. The major product of the collaboration is the Cochrane Database of Systematic Reviews of healthcare interventions which is published quarterly as part of the Cochrane Library. This database lists thousands of randomized controlled trials, and has conducted hundreds of meta-analyses on these trials, a number of which are directly relevant to MS.

The National Institute for Clinical Excellence

http://www.nice.org.uk

In the United Kingdom, the National Institute for Clinical Excellence provides detailed guidance on the management of a range of conditions, which includes MS. A key document in MS is *Guidelines on the management of multiple sclerosis in primary and secondary care* (2003)[1] which is available in downloadable pdf format from this website. This is an invaluable resource for all those affected by MS, and involved in the care of people with MS.

The NICE website also houses NICE published technology appraisals, which includes the appraisal on using beta interferon and glatiramer acetate in the treatment of multiple sclerosis.

The NHS Health Technology Assessment (HTA) Programme

http://www.hta.nhsweb.nhs.uk/

The aim of this programme is to provide all those who make decisions in the NHS with high-quality information on the costs, effectiveness, and broader impact of health care treatments and tests. These publications are freely available in CD-ROM format; or printed versions can be purchased. Those currently published specific to MS include:

- A cost-utility analysis of interferon beta.
- A systematic review of disease-modifying drugs.
- A systematic review for fatigue in multiple sclerosis.
- An evaluation of the role of MS specialist nurses.
- A review of the natural history and epidemiology of MS.
- A systematic review of treatments for spasticity and pain.
- The development of a patient-based measure of outcome in MS.

---

1 *Multiple sclerosis: management of multiple sclerosis in primary and secondary care.* Clinical Guidelines 8, National Institute for Clinical Excellence, November 2003.

Sources of information about practical issues relevant to living with MS

The Disabled Living Foundation (DLF)

http://www.dlf.org.uk/

The main aim of the DLF is to help older and disabled people find equipment solutions that enable them to lead independent lives. This site provides a range of information for members of the public and professionals, which includes:

- Downloadable fact sheets, providing advice on a wealth of topics including choosing equipment related to mobility, moving and handling, clothing and footwear, telecoms and alarms.
- Details re: suppliers of equipment.
- Discussion forums which facilitate discussion between users on equipment.
- A database for professionals to access information on over 14,000 items of equipment and their suppliers.

Ability Net

http://www.abilitynet.org.uk/

Ability Net aims to advise people on specialist assistive information technology, for any disability. Advice is available via its helpline and website. Factsheets are available to download, which give detailed information on a wide range of assistive technology services and organizations relevant to information technology.

Resources relevant to carers

- ACE National: *www.acecarers.org.uk*
- Carers information: *www.carersinformation.org.uk*
- Carers UK: *www.carersonline.org.uk*
- Carersline: 0808 808 7777
- Princess Royal Trust for Carers: *www.carers.org*

Resources relevant to families

- Contact a Family helpline: 0808 808 3555
- Contact a Family website: *www.cafamily.org.uk*
- Working Families: *www.parentsatwork.org.uk*
- MS Trust publications, which include *My Mum has MS*, *My Dad has MS*, and *The Young Persons guide to MS*. Available on *www.mstrust.org.uk*. This site also provides access to information and support.
- MS Society, which provides access to information, advice and support: *www.mssociety.org.uk*
- Relate: *www.relate.org.uk*
- Disability living Foundation: *www.dlf.org.uk*
- Disabled Parents Network: *www.disabledparentsnetwork.org.uk*
- The National MS Society publications directly relevant to young people include: *Keep S'myelin*, and *Teen Inside MS*. These are available on *www.nmss.org-American*
- Canadian MS Society has up to date information and an interactive activity section for young people with a parent with MS. Available on: *www.mssociety.ca*

Index